GEOGR
METHOДЅ ГОК
HEALTH SERVICES
RESEARCH

A Focus on the Rural – Urban Continuum

Edited by
THOMAS C. RICKETTS
LUCY A. SAVITZ
WILBERT M. GESLER*
DIANA N. OSBORNE

Cecil G. Sheps Center for Health Services Research
University of North Carolina at Chapel Hill

*Department of Geography
University of North Carolina at Chapel Hill

UNIVERSITY
PRESS OF
AMERICA

Lanham • New York • London

Library of Congress Cataloging-in-Publication Data

Geographic methods for health services research : a focus on the
rural-urban continuum / edited by Thomas C. Ricketts . . . [et al.].
        p.   cm.
Includes bibliographical references and index.
1. Rural health services—Resarch—Methodology.   2. Rural health
    services—Maps.   3. Medical geography—Methodology.
4. Medical geography—Maps.   5. Rural health services—United
States—Research—Methodology.   6. Rural health services—United
    States—Maps.   7. Medical geography—United States—
Methodology.   8. Medical geography—United States—Maps.
                    I. Ricketts, Thomas C.
    RA771.G46   1994   362.1'0425—dc20   94–9023 CIP

            ISBN 0–8191–9532–4 (cloth : alk. paper)
            ISBN 0–8191–9533–2 (pbk. : alk. paper)

Contents

List of Figures and Tables

Chapter 2
Focus on Rural and Regional Health Care Delivery
Figures

Chapter 3
Changes and Measures in the Crucial Dimension of Population

Chapter 4
Access to Health Services
Figures

Tables

Chapter 5
Health Professions Distribution
Figures

Tables

Chapter 6

Regionalization of Health Care

Figures

Tables

Chapter 7

Methods for Defining Medical Service Areas

Figures

Tables

Chapter 8

Contagious Diseases

Figures

Chapter 9
Evaluating Clusters of Adverse Health Outcomes
Figures

Preface

This book represents the third in a series of publications joining geography and rural health. In 1991, the North Carolina Rural Health Research Program, in the Cecil G. Sheps Center for Health Services Research at the University of North Carolina at Chapel Hill (UNC-CH), published the *National Rural Health Policy Atlas* with support from the US Office of Rural Health Policy. During the compilation of the *Atlas*, Wilbert M. Gesler, Ph.D., of the UNC-CH Department of Geography, and Thomas C. Ricketts, Ph.D., Director of the NC Rural Health Research Program, edited a collection of studies entitled *Health in Rural North America: The Geography of Health Care Services and Delivery*, which was published in 1992 by Rutgers University Press. *Geographic Methods for Health Services Research* is meant to complement these earlier works by offering interested practitioners, analysts, and policy makers access to the tools of geographic analysis, with special attention given to the issues relevant to rural health care.

The combination of rural health and geography is a natural extension of the long-standing interests of researchers in both the Department of Geography and the Sheps Center. John Florin, Ph.D., now Chair of the Geography Department at UNC-CH, had collaborated with staff of what was then the Health Services Research Center in the assessment of alternative configurations of the Health Service Areas (HSAs) in North Carolina as part of the development of the State's Health Planning and Development Agency. These cartographic analyses were the first to make use of hospital patient origin data, then maintained by the Center, and laid the groundwork for successive studies of patient origin at the Center. Edward Brooks, Dr.P.H., formerly the Associate Director of the Center, coordinated this work, which resulted in the publication of the monograph entitled "Strategic Directions for Health Planning in North Carolina" by the Center. The recommendations in that volume were incorporated into the State Health Plan as the HSA structure for North Carolina.

In the late 1970's, Thomas R. Konrad, Ph.D., Conrad Seipp, Ph.D., and John Florin, Ph.D. discussed the possibility of developing an atlas of health care and health care policy for the United States. A formal application was made to the National Center for Health Services Research in 1981 and modified proposals for an atlas of health care in North Carolina followed. These proposals were not funded but the interest in the use of geographic methods and cartographic displays was continually fostered within the Center. With the funding of the NC Rural Health Research Program in 1988 by the US Office of Rural Health Policy, the first real support for the compilation and production of an atlas spurred the interest of other faculty in the Department of Geography; Melinda Meade, Ph.D. and Wil Gesler, Ph.D. joined the group working on the *National Rural Health Policy Atlas*, contributing much of the text and interpretation. The rapidly developing field of desktop cartography allowed the *Atlas* to be completed without expensive investment in mainframe computer systems.

As the mapping capacity in the Center grew, requests for advice and technical assistance on geographic analysis began to come to the Center and the NC Rural Health Research Program. These requests ranged from the need for a simple description of rural versus urban counties to complex analyses of patient use patterns and the development of service area and activity space formulae for projects. The research team in the Rural Program and the Geography Department saw the need for a general introduction to the use of geography and cartography in health services research—especially in the field of rural health services in which spatial implications are a part of every issue. This need resulted in the submission of a proposal to the US Agency for Health Care Policy and Research to develop this book. We feel that *Geographic Methods for Health Services Research* meets the needs of researchers and policy makers alike by providing an introduction to basic and applied geographic terms and describing several of the most useful geographic analytic techniques. These are tools which can help us understand the problems involved in health care delivery in both urban and rural places.

Acknowledgments

This book would not have been published without the support of a grant by the US Agency for Health Care Policy and Research for the project entitled, "Preparation of a Geographical Study of Rural Health," Grant Number HS06706-02, Thomas C. Ricketts, Ph.D., Principal Investigator and Wilbert M. Gesler, Ph.D., Co-Investigator. We would like to acknowledge the patience and support of the Project Officer for that grant, Jean Carmody, M.S.W., who gave numerous constructive suggestions for the book and arranged for its external review. We would also like to thank the three anonymous reviewers who gave many useful suggestions and corrected several errors. Any remaining errors are the responsibility of the editors. We would like to acknowledge the support of the US Office of Rural Health Policy and its grant to the Cecil G. Sheps Center for Health Services Research of the University of North Carolina at Chapel Hill for the North Carolina Rural Health Research Program, Grant Number CSR000002-02-0, and the Project Officer for that grant, Patricia Taylor, Ph.D. Much of the development of the geographic analysis system used in the construction of the book was supported by that grant. Lastly, we would like to thank the Director, Gordon H. DeFriese, Ph.D., and the staff of the Cecil G. Sheps Center for their support and encouragement while the book was being written and put into final form.

Thomas C. Ricketts
Lucy A. Savitz
Wilbert M. Gesler
Diana N. Osborne

Chapter 1

Introduction

A Bit of Background

This work began as a geography of rural health in America. Our primary aim was twofold—to compile a cartographic presentation of major rural health issues, and to demonstrate how rural health care issues can be illustrated and analyzed using geographic and cartographic techniques and methods. As we continued our work, we were increasingly struck by the gap between the development and use of these approaches by academic geographers and the paucity of their use in health care planning and policy decisions. It was sensed that the greater need was to provide a sort of handbook that would help health care planners and professionals in both rural and urban settings better understand the nature and applicability of methods of geographic analysis to their problems. The result is this book. We have not lost our focus on the special problems facing rural America. However, the changing landscape in the United States dictates that our focus broaden to one of the rural–urban continuum. A clear dichotomy has ceased to exist. Many of our examples are drawn from rural conditions, and all of the methods can be used in a rural context.

Goals

While the use of geography and cartographic techniques in the analysis of health services access and health planning is growing, most policy decisions that have a direct relationship to the geographic allocation of health care services have been made without the active involvement of geographers or geographic analysis. These decisions include the various health planning and regionalization plans adopted in the US over the past half-century, the redistribution of manpower and facilities through legislation or regulation, and areal differentials in charge and fee levels. All of these decisions could benefit from the use of appropriate geographic analyses.

Though many of the problems relating to the unequal distribution of health care resources across the United States have long been recognized, it is only recently that a major effort has been made to ameliorate that distribution. Rural health problems that are intimately linked with the geography of the country include inequities in the distribution of health manpower and facilities, barriers to accessibility and utilization of health services, unequal benefits from federal health financing programs, lower health status for residents of some areas, the urban focus of the regionalization of many health delivery and provider systems, and the concentration of some high-risk populations in rural areas.

Geographic analysis of ecological patterns, and of changes in those patterns, can aid understanding of disease distribution and associations. The landscape that distinguishes a place is a complex expression of physical, biotic, and cultural processes. When one knows how to analyze its elements and patterns, one can usually determine what diseases might be found there. This is true at every scale, from a house and its backyard to the international landscape of the global economy. As populations grow and the economy changes, landscapes are altered in ways that may increase disease risk or enhance protection from it. The complex interactions between populations, behavior, and the physical environment comprise disease systems, and development can and does create change in those systems. Many of these patterns vary across the rural–urban continuum, and their locational context is important. Rocky Mountain spotted fever, for example, is a disease of the suburban–rural fringe, and its geography has changed as the suburbs invade rural America. AIDS has often been thought of as an urban problem in this country, but it is spreading to rural areas; the delay in the development of rural incidence relates to the general pattern of the spread of infectious disease. Health services delivery and disease ecology use similar evaluative techniques. This sharing of method will benefit both aspects of research and inquiry.

This book is meant to guide a variety of users in the application of analytic geography and cartographic techniques to health policy analysis and health services research, with a focus upon rural communities and populations. It demonstrates these applications within the context of problems encountered in the analysis of the distribution of disease, various health indicators, and health care resources that have direct relevance to rural communities and rural populations. These problems are not, however, restricted to rural America, since the health care system integrates services, programs, and institutions from all parts of the country across the rural–urban continuum. Indeed, it is difficult in modern America to clearly define and dichotomize the two (see Chapter 2). The concerns of rural and urban America, as well as their geography, are intertwined.

This book is intended as a starting point. It should serve as a source book of tools for planners in the field and a guide for users of geographic data. It is aimed at a variety of audiences including:

1. Government planners at all levels, who may adapt the methods and techniques to their own particular problems.

2. Policy analysts, who could use the techniques as alternative ways to examine and display data.

3. Policy makers, who might use the handbook to assist them in understanding how to interpret and analyze geographic data and suggest solutions to health services delivery and allocation problems.

4. Health care facility managers and organizational planners, who could use these techniques to develop operations and marketing programs for their institutions.

5. Physicians and clinicians, who might use these analytic approaches to identify their patient populations and in planning community-based interventions.

6. Academic geographers, who should find the book useful as a text to illustrate methods and introduce issues in health services research.

It is the authors' hope that this book can and will be used by planners, health professionals, and geographers. Most of the methods and techniques introduced here do not demand either sophisticated computer hardware or software, nor do they require a substantial background in either geography or statistics. The health care issues we have selected as examples are mostly common ones that must be dealt with by many providers and planners across the rural–urban continuum. Throughout the text we touch upon other issues that might be addressed within the same or a similar conceptual or methodological framework as a way of suggesting the broad utility of many of our approaches. We are confident that the user can identify other appropriate applications.

Health Problems of Rural America

Rural America stands in poor contrast to urban and suburban parts of the country with regard to health status and health care resources. This condition mirrors the relative status of rural populations in wealth, education, and employment. In health care, nonmetropolitan counties in the United States, in 1984, had 26 percent of the country's poor but only 13.5 percent of the physicians. As of 1990, although 22.5 percent of the US population lived in nonmetropolitan areas, only 13.2 percent of all patient care physicians and 6.7 percent of hospital-based physicians were practicing in those areas. Rural residents report lower health status although they are more likely to be hospitalized, and report seeing physicians at approximately the same rate as their urban counterparts. This may be because of higher rates of chronic disease, especially among the rural elderly. Infant mortality in rural communities is higher than in urban areas for all races, with the highest rates encountered in nonmetropolitan counties in the Southeast. Rural accident rates are high. Rural hospitals have been closing at an alarming rate and trends in the distribution of physicians and clinics in rural communities appear to be reversing the growth patterns of the 70's and early 80's. Rural residents are less likely than their urban counterparts to be insured for their health care costs, especially by private insurance. Additionally, an estimated four million rural Americans are migrant and seasonal farmworkers. Their numbers create a series of special rural health problems. Migrant workers (perhaps a third of the four million) have a variety of health problems, including ailments associated with overcrowding and poor sanitary living conditions, a high rate of parasitic infections, poor nutrition, and acute and chronic illnesses related to pesticide use.

Medical Geography

Medical geography uses the concepts and techniques of geography to investigate health-related topics. The discipline has an ancient perspective. Hippocrates, in *On Airs, Waters, and Places*, wrote nearly 2,500 years ago that:

> Whoever wishes to investigate medicine properly, should proceed thus: in the first place to consider the seasons of the year, and what effects each of them produces. … We must also consider the qualities of the waters, for as they differ from one another in taste and weight, so do they differ much in their qualities. In the same manner, when one comes into a city to which he is a stranger, he ought to consider its situation, how it lies as to the winds and the rising of the sun; for its influence is not the same whether it lies to the north or the south, to the rising or setting sun. These things one ought to consider most attentively, …

This ecological perspective on the nature of health and disease remained dominant in Western thinking until the development of germ theory in the 19th century. For 2,000 years Western medicine maintained this central concern for geographic variations in nearly every aspect of the physical and human world.

The term "medical geography" was apparently first introduced by 18th and 19th century physicians working in this same tradition. One such physician was Dr. John Snow. He contended cholera was a water-borne disease, and that the source of an 1854 London epidemic of the disease could be traced to the city's public wells. Snow constructed a dot map of locations of all of the identified cholera cases in the city. His map demonstrated a clear concentration of cases around the Broad Street well. Snow encouraged local authorities to remove the pump handle from the well, which they did. Although cholera incidence had declined prior to the removal of the handle, the role of disease mapping in public health was firmly established after Snow published his results focusing on the role of the map.

Effective cartography and map interpretation have been impor-tant elements in the evolution of modern medical geography. A milestone in this development was the *World Atlas of Epidemic Diseases*, published in ten parts in Germany between 1952 and 1961 under the editorship of H. L. Jusatz. These maps were perhaps the first attempt to present medical facts about disease occurrence along with associated environmental conditions on a single map. At about the same time Jacques May, working in the United States, presented a series of disease maps in his *The Ecology of Human Disease* (1958). More recently, national atlases of mortality have been published in Japan, Great Britain, and other countries. Excellent atlases of cancer mortality are available for China and the United States. British geographers Andrew Cliff and Peter Haggett have provided a magnificent overview of the problems and possibilities inherent to medical cartography in their *Atlas of Disease Distribu-tions* (1988). Meade, Florin, and Gesler have provided a compre-hensive survey of modern medical geography in their *Medical Geography* (1988).

Atlases present the products of the application of certain geo-graphic and cartographic analyses; this book presents steps that lead to maps and displays that can be used in policy analysis or research.

Organization

Early chapters of the book deal with general issues relating to the examination of health care in rural areas; later chapters move on to more specific issues as they relate to health care delivery and health policy. Points of Departure are included with the chapters to provide more detailed information about some of the points raised in the text.

Chapter 2, *A Focus on Rural and Regional Health Care Delivery*, examines the concept and definitions of "rural," with a special focus on the geographic interpretation of the term. We discuss rurality as it relates to health care, health policy analysis, and health services research. The chapter concludes with a model that presents the relationship between transportation and health services along the rural–urban continuum. The Point of Departure, *Issues Related to Population Density*, describes the importance of population density in characterizing any spatial area and in provision and placement of health care services.

In Chapter 3, *Changes and Measures in the Crucial Dimension of Population*, we first recognize that demographically there are different types of rural areas, and that these different population structures suggest the need for different approaches to the provision of health services. The chapter examines the effects of age and migration, and the use and analysis of such demographic techniques as small area analysis, demographic base maps, population potential maps, social activity cells, locational quotients, and population pyramids; use of censuses of population, business, and agriculture is also discussed. *Data Sources for Health Services Research* is the Point of Departure accompanying this chapter, and provides general guidance for readers on issues concerning the acquisition and use of secondary data. Also included is a list of contacts for help in obtaining the data required to conduct various analyses described throughout the text.

Chapter 4, *Access to Health Services*, begins with a discussion of access as a concept with respect to how it has been addressed in the literature. This discussion takes the reader one step further by introducing a framework by which access is viewed as coverage. Geographic considerations pertinent to this discussion as well as basic measures of access are introduced. The chapter concludes with a brief overview of emerging questions in access and a Point of Departure, *Access and Cartography*, that emphasizes the application of cartography in examining access to health care.

Chapter 5, *Health Professions Distributions*, emphasizes the geographic availability of health care. Specifically, it teases out the associated issues of availability and equity. The example of the distribution of various types of oncologists in North Carolina is used as a case study to examine those issues. This chapter also presents a variety of methods for measuring availability and equity, the assessment of supply and demand, and the importance of the proper scale of geographic analysis. Two Points of Departure are provided to further elucidate topics raised in the chapter: *Community-Based Measures of Underservice*, and *Tracking Doctors into the Twenty-First Century*.

Chapter 6, *Regionalization of Health Care*, begins with a review of the concept of health care regionalization and a brief look at a number of earlier regionalization efforts in North Carolina. We emphasize in the chapter that different regional schemes may be appropriate for different specific purposes. The most appropriate regionalization for a given situation must incorporate differences in geographic scale, available resources, areal patterns of need, and patterns of transportation and human movement. Regions can be created based on the rural–urban continuum, hierarchical arrangements, labor market areas, and cluster analysis. They can be used for many purposes, including the identification of hospital service areas (using flow maps), or the designation of service areas for clinic programs. *Rural Places and Regionalization* and *Geographic Information Systems (GIS)* are Points of Departure developed to expand the discussion of these topics beyond that provided within the chapter.

Chapter 7, *Methods for Defining Medical Service Areas*, provides the background and context for identifying medical service areas. Several methods are examined and compared through a concise literature review, and descriptions of different methodologies along with figures depicting them. The chapter concludes with a list of factors to be considered when selecting a service area methodology, and provides three examples of the use of these factors in choosing a methodology appropriate to a specific research aim. The chapter concludes with a Point of Departure entitled *Hospital Closure and Access to Hospital Services*, which depicts use of a geographic method to project market reassignment based on consumer behavior following hospital closure.

Chapter 8, *Contagious Diseases*, focuses on the factors involved in the geographic diffusion of contagious diseases; the distribution of HIV and tuberculosis in North Carolina are used as examples. The significant role of the return migration of AIDS patients from out-of-state, often from AIDS epicenters, identifies a series of HIV-related issues for rural areas. The tuberculosis discussion utilizes data from a survey of farm workers in North Carolina. We discuss conditions affecting the spread of disease with regard to migrant camps and patterns of activity; choropleth maps of TB incidence/prevalence rates are used to fill out this discussion. The Point of Departure with this chapter, *Adjustment of Tuberculosis Incidence Rates*, provides a clear discussion of the merits of adjusted vs. unadjusted incidence rates, the need for rate adjustment, particularly for comparison purposes, and techniques used in adjusting rates.

The focus of Chapter 9, *Evaluating Clusters of Adverse Health Outcomes*, is on problems associated with data availability and appropriate denominators needed to identify cancer clusters, and on methods of measuring cluster significance. Three different examples drawn from North Carolina are used to illustrate difficulties inherent in the identification process, as well as the potential role in this process of Geographic Information Systems (GIS). The Point of Departure included in this final chapter is *State Cancer Control Map and Data Program Analyses*. It describes a computer program that allows examination of cancer data at the state level, and can produce both tabular and cartographic displays of these data.

We conclude with a *Glossary of Technical Terms* and *Technical Notes*. Terminology can often be a barrier to effective communication. Readers may be unfamiliar with many of the terms used throughout this book; the Glossary should provide insight on these terms. The

Technical Notes provide general information on issues to do with cartography and graphic representations of data. Also included in the Technical Notes is a list of various software packages, many of which were used in the analyses and figures included in this book. We have by no means tried to provide a complete list; rather, we give an overview of what we have used, provide address information for specific software vendors, and indicate where to locate more exhaustive listings of available software.

Chapter 2

A Focus on Rural and Regional Health Care Delivery

Point of Departure:
Population Density and Research

Introduction

One of the most vexing problems in health care delivery in the United States is how to provide an adequate level of health care services to rural populations. Rural Americans have long been at a disadvantage in gaining access to basic primary care services, much less specialty services, because medical care resources tend to concentrate themselves in urban or suburban places.

Public policy interest in the special problems of rural health care has fluctuated over time. When interest is high, or when new programs have been mounted to address these problems, the field of health services research seems to take greater notice as well. The number of conferences convened during the late 1980's to address rural issues, the funding of rural health research centers and the US Office of Rural Health Policy by the Congress, and the initiation of rural outreach and rural hospital transition grant programs in the Health Resources and Services Administration (HRSA) and the Health Care Financing Administration (HCFA) are reflections of the current concern in the Congress and in the States over the severe shortages of qualified health care personnel in rural communities and the financial plight of certain small rural hospitals and other health care facilities.

The focus of this book is on methods of geographic analysis in health services research, but the context in which we describe these methods and the examples we provide concentrate on rural issues and the problems of rural populations. The use of geographic approaches and concepts in the study of rural health services is very appropriate because rurality is itself primarily a geographic expression, and because of the continuing concern with access to services for rural populations. The examples are not confined to rural situations although much current interest in health care delivery focuses on rural underserved populations and their problems of access. The dominant barrier to access to health care for rural underserved populations is geographic in nature. This chapter discusses the "rural" nature of communities as a means of understanding the utilization of services in conjunction with the apparent health status of populations, rather than to make a point that "rural" places are more or less further along a continuum of place types.

In this book we are not concerned with the question of "what is rural," we talk instead about a continuum in the American landscape that can best be understood as an integrated or regional concept that recognizes the relationships and dependencies between urban and rural places. This concept is appropriate in research because urban and rural comparisons often call for a hierarchical characterization in health services. A separate "rural health" concept may have a precarious existence in the future. We may be more concerned with regional and coordinated systems than with making distinctions between cities and farms if regional networks are implemented.

We will consider gradations and relations between urban centers, the suburban rings, small towns, and the very rural and frontier places in the United States. It is vital to remember that health care services are seldom self-sufficient in a rural place or small town. There are many operating ties between urban tertiary care systems and the rural practitioner and patient. As a geographic concept using a continuum is more helpful in analyses than is a strict rural–urban contrast, particularly when data are used to describe the processes and structures that make up the health care system.

Health Services Research
and Rural America

There was great interest in the problem of physician specialty and geographic provider maldistribution in the 1960's and 1970's. Ratio analysis and descriptive studies of supply showed a major shift toward specialty medicine and a drop in the numbers of physicians setting up practice in rural and nonmetropolitan areas. These early studies of health professional supply and specialty mix became more sophisticated as mathematical models for specific practitioner need and supply were developed by the Bureau of Health Manpower in the US Department of Health, Education and Welfare (US Bureau of Health Manpower, 1977). These models examined the national supply of providers and pointed clearly to trends in which specialists would dominate the system and most practitioners would locate in urban places. The methods for forecasting supply and need were very well-developed and docu-mented, allowing those interested in replicating the analyses or targeting them for selected states and regions to do so easily (Kriesberg et al., 1976). Individual communities were not the early target of health professions need and supply studies until the federal government implemented programs to build local capacity, such as the National Health Service Corps (NHSC) and the Neighborhood, later Community Health Centers (CHC) programs. These initia-tives required the development of methods to identify underserved communities in which to locate programs and providers. The development of appropriate criteria was long and involved and no completely satisfactory approach was found (Ricketts & Pathman, 1991). In the end, the designation of areas which were underserved rested primarily on the ratio of physicians-to-population for US counties; those counties in the bottom fourth of the distribution of ratios were considered "underserved" and, thus, eligible for program support. The definition currently in use is a direct descendent of that ratio method with modifications for high-risk populations. Under current regulations, Health Professions Shortage Areas (HPSAs) can be whole counties, groups of Census tracts, specific populations (e.g., migrants or indigents), or institutions (e.g., prisons).

There was concern during this period that simple physician-to-population ratios were inadequate measures of health care requirements, and that they oversimplified the real picture of need while failing to incorporate actual use of services (Jeffers, Bognanno & Bartlett, 1971). Various efforts were made to estimate the "need" or "demand" for physician services in small geographic areas, usually counties, and to relate these estimates to available data on the current supply of such practitioners, but none could be translated into workable policies.

Provider Supply in Rural Areas

Specific geographic studies of the distribution of providers, with a focus on their presence in rural areas, were completed by the RAND Corporation in the early 1980's. Researchers at the RAND Corporation used the American Medical Association's Physician Masterfile data to examine the flow of physicians, by specialty, into nonmetropolitan areas (Schwartz, Newhouse, Bennett & Williams, 1980). This first study by the RAND group found that from 1960 to 1977 the absolute increase in the number of specialists per 100,000 population in eight clinical disciplines was greater in metropolitan areas, but the percentage increase remained higher in small towns, where the smallest towns studied were communities of 2,500 population. Hence, those communities with the most severe access problems may have been excluded from consideration.

This study was followed by another by the same authors, showing that nearly every town with a population of more than

2,500 people in 1979 had a physician in active medical practice in some specialty (Newhouse, Williams, Bennett & Schwartz, 1982). The third study by the RAND group (Williams, Schwartz, Newhouse & Bennett, 1983) developed a quite different database which included calculations of the straight-line geographic distances from the centers of population in all communities of less than 25,000 population to the geographic locations of all actively practicing physicians in all specialties for 16 states. These distances were converted to highway miles through a special procedure developed and validated especially for this research. The study found that the road distances rural residents had to travel to all types of medical specialists had decreased in the period from 1970 to 1979, and, as the total number of general practice and family practice physicians decreased, physicians in other medical specialties tended to take up practice in places where generalists were once the sole type of practitioner. Ninety-six percent of the rural populations they studied lived within 15 miles of some type of physician. From an examination of the volume of new physicians expected to be graduated from American medical schools and medical residency training programs, the RAND group predicted that this trend would certainly continue. This study lent support to the so-called "trickle-down," "sandpile," or "diffusion" theory of physician manpower distribution.

Collectively, these papers argued that the overall volume of new physicians produced by the nation's medical schools and residency programs was effectively ensuring a reasonable level of geographic accessibility to some type of physician care, although a person in some of these small communities might not be able to access a physician in a specialty of his/her choice within these same geographic distances. As a result, there may have to be some degree of "substitutability" among physician types for persons who live in these locations.

The RAND studies have been highly controversial (Kindig & Movassaghi, 1989; Budetti, 1984; Fruen & Cantwell, 1982). The criticisms pointed out that the crow-fly method used to calculate distances did not reflect the reality of travel to physicians, that the proximity to a physician does not reflect the actual availability of services, that a substantial portion of the physicians included in the calculation were not practicing full-time, and that the sample of states examined did not include some of the worst examples of geographic inaccessibility. Newhouse (1990) responded to some of the criticism these papers have received, arguing that much of the controversy has arisen from both a theoretical misunderstanding of the economic theory these studies were designed to test and from a misinterpretation of the empirical data presented in the papers. In a lengthy discussion of the economic location theory upon which the work of the RAND group was based, Newhouse shows that the notion depicted in the use of the "trickle-down" label is inaccurate and inappropriate. The theory actually describes what Newhouse would define as a trend toward "spreading out" the available physician supply among a number of practice location options. The choice of specific location has far more to do with the general economic context than it does with the size of the community. He argues that as more physicians consider nonmetropolitan practice locations, they are likely to choose to locate in communities already served by practicing physicians, since they will want to maximize their own demand and will view the prior location of other physicians as an important indication of patterns of consumer behavior.

Newhouse's line of thinking bears remarkable resemblance to the pattern of settlement of a sample of 900 young physicians between 1973 and 1976. Most who located in communities of less than 10,000 population tended to settle in communities where there was already a medical community of one or more other doctors (Madison & Combs, 1981). Sixty-seven percent of these doctors tended to locate in communities where there were four or more other doctors already in practice. Only seven percent located in communities where they would be the only physician. Moreover, Madison and Combs found that a much lower percentage of physicians in their sample were likely to choose the smallest communities when compared with the choices made by physicians subsidized by private foundations and government agencies.

The study of the supply of providers in rural versus urban communities and the development of indices of need continue to be important in rural health services research. Policy and funding initiatives exist to promote training of rural practitioners and primary care providers, including the funding of the Rural Interdisciplinary Health Team Training Program in the Bureau of Health Professions, the Practice Sights: State Primary Care Development Strategies program of the Robert Wood Johnson Foundation, and the continued publication of comprehensive studies of rural health professions distribution (US Office of Technology Assessment, 1990; Kindig, Schmelzer & Hong, 1992; Study of models, 1992).

Rural Hospitals

Another main area of concern in rural health services research is utilization and survival of the rural hospital. During the second half of the 1980's, small rural hospitals began to close at an increasing rate (Mullner & McNeil, 1986). Urban hospitals were also closing but at a slower rate (US OTA, 1990). The reasons for the high failure rate of rural hospitals were debated but, in the minds of the administrators and advocates for rural health, lay squarely at the feet of the Prospective Payment System changes implemented in the first half of the 1980's. Spokespersons for rural hospitals claimed that payment differentials between urban and rural hospitals created the conditions that broke the backs of the hospitals that closed (National Rural Health Association, 1991). Congress and the Health Care Financing Administration responded with modifications in the regulations that created special classes of rural hospitals, the rural referral center and the sole community hospital, and eventually closed the payment gap between the two groups. Numerous studies were commissioned by the Prospective Payment Assessment Commission and the Health Care Financing Administration to study the problems facing rural hospitals. These studies used varying measures of rurality based upon the changing definitions of a rural hospital or rural populations that were included in legislation. The central questions being asked were: Did rural residents have lower access to care when hospitals closed? and, Did rural residents bypass rural hospitals to use urban hospitals?

The driving issue behind health services research focusing on rural populations was access to services, and many studies analyzed evidence that rural residents had either restricted or potentially lower levels of access when compared to either urban residents or some national standard. The policy application of the results of this research led to legislation and programs which targeted rural populations or made exceptions for rural communities. As these programs were implemented, it became apparent that more useful definitions of rurality and rural places were needed. This spurred interest in the question, "What is rural?".

Rurality and Concepts of Rurality

There is no universally accepted definition of "rural." Rural sociologists have debated the definition and no clear consensus has been attained (Willits, Bealer & Timbers, 1990). The "ideal" of rurality in the United States is tied to the traditions and collective identity of Americans who saw and see rural places as part of the "garden" where people are honest, religious, individualistic, and hard workers who lead simple lives (Marx, 1964). Rural America has never been completely agricultural and never completely synonymous with agriculture since the nation encompasses desert, tundra, swamp, and mountainous terrain as well as arable plains, valleys, and piedmont. In contrast with the extreme variety in the landscape across rural communities, we see that there is a unity of perception of rural-ness that reflects the ideal embodied in a symbol like "small-town America," whether the dominant industry in that town is mining, farming, tourism, or light industry. These "images" of rural life are used again and again in America for purposes as disparate as the development of local identity and pride to the construction of an abstract vision of by-gone days to help sell off-road vehicles to urban accountants. The popular images have been distilled into five general types by rural sociologists (Miller & Luloff, 1981):

> 1. Positive images of rural life: characterized by statements like: "brings out the best in people—makes for close knit families—friendly and neighborly—peace and quiet";

2. Negative images of rural life: "monotonous and boring—provincial and narrow minded thinking—crude and uncultured in manners and dress—no opportunities to get ahead—doing without the good things";

3. Anti-urban sentiment: "urban living is too fast and dangerous—urban life is centered on money and consumption—impersonal and uncaring";

4. Agrarian values: "agriculture is natural—the family farm is the backbone of American democracy—the farm is the best place for a family";

5. Wilderness values: "open areas are good and healthy places—solitude brings peace—wilderness is an important part of our national heritage."

These characterizations help to distill our assumptions and biases concerning rural America but they do not directly contribute to our understanding of why rural life would be associated with differences in medical care and health status. A system proposed by Wibberly (Wibberly, 1972) and supported by Miller and Luloff (1981) relates some fundamental characteristics of rural populations to health services. That system, in modified form, is presented in Table 2-1. These basic, physical characteristics of rural places and people have implications for health services, but they are used most often to explain observed phenomena rather than to organize hypotheses or structure a system of knowledge to understand rural health.

These characterizations of rurality allow us to classify rural health services research into six areas that nearly parallel the concepts described above. Examples of health services research that fall into each category are included in the section later in this chapter on *The Rural–Urban Continuum and Health Services Research*.

Table 2-1

Rural Characteristics and Health Services Implications

Rural Characterization	Health Services Implication	Contrast Concept
1. Use of the land	Agricultural injuries, occupational injury rates.	Little dependence upon the land in occupational illness.
2. Delimited area	Service area, market area dependent upon urban, central places, carrying capacity of population for hierarchy of professionals and technologies.	No boundaries, definition by other characteristics, e.g. race, age.
3. Small population	Occurrence of disease is masked by small numbers, calculation of rates is difficult. Limited financial base to support resources, need for regionalization.	Large populations allow for understanding rates and identifying problems. No problems with financial support.
4. Dispersed population	Travel time to services, travel time to patients, communications needs.	Concentrated population.
5. Identity as countryside	Rural attitudes toward medicine and health care, independence, neighborliness, structure of health problems related to social and economic characteristics.	No unifying identity (suburbs) or urban identity.
6. Isolation from technology	Late innovation, travel time greater to technology, provider isolation.	Closely linked to technology transfer, no lag in innovation.

Source: Adapted from Wibberly GP. 1972. Conflicts in the countryside. *Town and Country Planning* 40:259-64.

Rural Health and Health Policy

Much of what has been written recently about rural places uses definitions based on a geographical standard using county or place size, focusing more on the diversity rather than the underlying characteristics of rurality (McGranahan et al., 1986). Whether or not there is a distinct notion of rural when it comes to health care services, we rarely see programs that take into consideration the special living patterns of rural people (Rowles, 1988). We more often see concern with the structure of services in rural communities or those serving rural communities. This "policy-oriented" approach is more one of perception of the rural landscape as containing this or that resource rather than the ways in which people use what they have (or don't have).

The identification of rural areas and populations for policy purposes usually depends upon boundary-setting and the ability to categorize if not dichotomize. The setting of boundaries causes problems in classification because there are so many existing geopolitical boundaries which are usually drawn for reasons other than the delimiting of rural versus other populations. They are set up for governmental reasons of all types including general governmental purposes (counties, townships, tax districts, boroughs) for specific services.

Rural can be seen as a positively derived concept, that is, one starts with defining what rural is, perhaps contrasting rural to urban or suburban or defining rural, and then saying that the rest is something else which others may define as urban. The opposite is to define urban or other categories of place and people and to leave the remainder as rural. The latter process is the approach of the US Bureau of the Census. Cities and places with 2,500 or more people are "urban" and the remainder are "rural." The same happens in the US Office of Management and Budget's classification of counties in the United States as metropolitan or nonmetropolitan. The former group meets certain criteria for size and market dominance and what is left are the nonmetro counties. These two governmental characterizations of the population essentially drive the comparison of populations and places as urban and rural; rural thereby is more of a "residual" than a unified concept. This may explain why many recent analysts have discovered such a great diversity in the nonmetropolitan counties of the country and why they have difficulty identifying simple or single policies to improve resource allocation in rural places. The most recent review of various scales and typologies was done by Hewitt (1989; 1992). These largely represent the hierarchies and classifications of economically-defined rurality. The same is true of the USDA classification of rural counties by primary mode of production or economic situation (persistent poverty, manufacturing, government, etc.).

Definitions of Rurality
and Health Policy

The way rurality is defined in the context of rural health policy and health policy in general has been described exhaustively by Maria Hewitt in her paper for the US Office of Technology Assessment (OTA), *Defining "Rural" Areas: Impact on Health Care Policy and Research* (1989) and in a subsequent summary and update to that work (Hewitt, 1992). This review and synthesis of definitions of rurality and how they affect health policy decisions was completed as part of the OTA's large-scale project examining health care in rural America. In her review, Hewitt described rurality in terms of government jurisdictions, mostly counties. She regarded this restriction as a drawback to precise studies of rural populations and health care. The two most common classification systems used in health policy are those of the US Office of Management and Budget (OMB) and the US Bureau of the Census.

The systems to classify counties that Hewitt reviews represent the extensive efforts on the part of analysts and researchers to make sense of the rural–urban continuum and to identify "types" of rural places. For example, the allocation of differential Medicare payments to rural hospitals must be based on some consistent definition of "rural" that relates to the policy purposes of the difference. It was assumed that rural hospitals had lower labor and capital costs due to less reliance on technology; the definition of rural should then identify those places where these conditions prevailed. The definition of rural applied here was initially hospitals outside of Metropolitan Statistical Areas or those serving rural populations. This definition caused a great deal of resentment among the rural hospitals who felt that this description did not reflect the reality of costs and that "rural" did not equate to lower costs. Figure 2-1 illustrates the overlap of populations using the Census and OMB designations—it is clear that not all rural populations are nonmetropolitan nor all urban people, metropolitan.

Figure 2-1
Rural-Urban-Metropolitan-Frontier, A Map Example

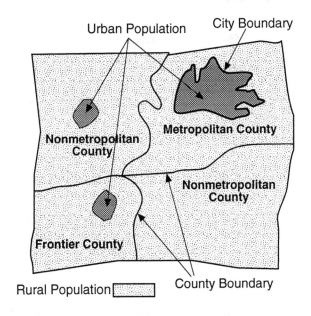

Comparing Classification Systems: Physicians in Rural America

Various categorizations of rurality have been used in analyses of the distribution of professionals, the diffusion of technology, comparative studies of disease rates and care patterns, and the distribution of resources. One system, proposed by the US Department of Agriculture and called the Rural–Urban Continuum for Metro and Non-Metro Counties (Butler, 1990), was used to track the distribution of US physicians from 1975 to 1988 (Frenzen, 1991). This classification scheme is based on county population and adjacency to a Metropolitan Statistical Area. The non-metro portion includes urbanized (20,000 or more urban residents), less urbanized (2,500 to 19,999 urban residents), and rural counties (less

Table 2-2
Rural and Urban Populations in Metro and Nonmetro
Counties, 1990 Census Data

	Metro	NonMetro	Total
Rural	26,525,155	35,133,175	61,658,330
	13.8%	62.7%	
Urban	166,201,175	20,850,368	187,051,543
	86.2%	37.3%	
Total	192,726,330	55,983,543	**248,709,873**

Source: US Bureau of the Census. 1990 Census, Summary Tape File 3C.
Washington, DC: Department of Commerce.

than 2,500 urban residents), then divides each of those into adjacent or nonadjacent subcategories. Frenzen analyzed physician-to-population ratios for each group of counties for 1975, 1981, and 1988 using data from the US Bureau of Health Professions and plotted the proportions of primary care and specialist MDs and all DOs per 100,000 population for each of the county categories. Figure 2-2 is adapted from those data. The horizontal axis emphasizes the notion that this categorization scheme is a continuum and represents a unified, linear description of the rurality of counties.

The American Medical Association (AMA) also classified counties on a continuum from the most urban to the most rural. The AMA system is based solely on Metropolitan Statistical Area (Standard Metropolitan Statistical Area [SMSA] when devised) designation and population. Fruen and Cantwell (1982) tracked primary care physician supply from 1950 through 1978 using this categorization. Their analysis using these classifications was a

Figure 2-2
Nonfederal MDs per 100,000 Population by USDA
Urban–Rural Continuum Category, 1975-1988

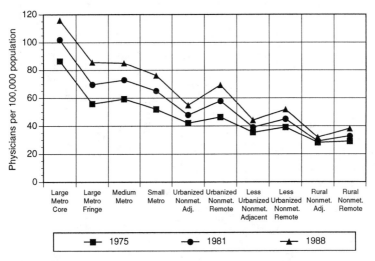

Source: Adapted from Frenzen PD. 1991. The increasing supply of physicians in US urban and rural areas, 1975 to 1988. *American Journal of Public Health* 81(9):1141-1147.

comparison of ratios of total population-to-primary care physicians in categories of metropolitan and nonmetropolitan counties for seven years: 1950, 1960, 1970, 1972, 1974, 1976 and 1978. Figure 2-3 is adapted from that analysis and shows 4 years of the data. The figure should not be compared directly with Figure 2-2 since the analysis tracks only changes in primary care physicians.

David Kindig and his associates have examined physician supply in the smallest rural counties in the United States and compared changes over time looking at absolute population size and population density (Kindig & Movassaghi, 1989). They have also used an alternative categorization of nonmetropolitan counties to examine physician distribution and use of services (Hong & Kindig, 1992). This system is based on the employment, commuting, and population characteristics of the counties and was proposed by Jerome Pickard (1988) of the Appalachian Regional Commis-

Figure 2-3
Primary Care Physicians per 100,000 Population,
AMA Classification System

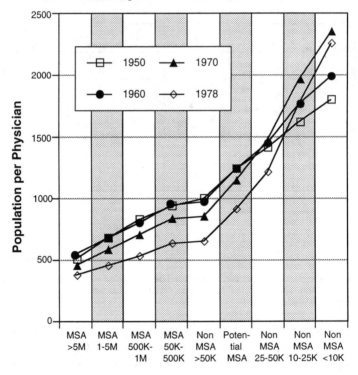

Source: Adapted from Fruen MA and JR Cantwell. 1982. Geographic distribution of physicians: Past trends and future influences. *Inquiry* 19(1):44-50.

sion. This classification system incorporates ratios of workers working in the county to those working outside the county drawn from Census figures: the percentage of the population working outside the county, the absolute number of urban residents, the proportion of total population that is urban, and the total population.

Table 2-3 describes the structure of the Pickard classification system and the 11 levels of classification. The system depends heavily on the employee-to-resident ratio (E/R) and the proportion of workers with their primary employment outside of the county.

Table 2-3
The Pickard Classification System

County type	E/R ratio	Percent of workers working out of county	Urban population	Percent of population urban	Total population
Metro centers	.98 or higher	< 30%			
Metro satellites	≥ .70 and ≤ .97	< 30%			
Metro commuting satellites	.70 or higher	≥ 30%			
Metro suburban	≥ .50 and ≤ .69				
Metro dormitory	< .50				
Nonmetro centers	.98 or higher OR .85 or higher	less than 30%	Place of 10,000 or more	25% or more	25,000 or more 10,000 or more
Nonmetro satellites: Does not qualify for Nonmetro center AND	.70 or higher	less than 30% and at least 15%	5,000 or more		10,000 or more
Nonmetro commuting with center: would qualify as n.m. center, n.m. satellite or n.m. small center but has more outcommuting		30% or more			
Nonmetro small centers: does not qualify for above, AND	≥1.20 OR ≥ .98 OR ≥ 0.85 and ≤ 0.97	less than 30%	2,000 or more If less than 3,500 must have ----->	20% or higher	2,000 or more
Rural commuting counties: Does not qualify for above but has more outcommuting than n.m. rural		30% or more			
Nonmetro rural: does not qualify for any other n.m. categories					

Source: Adapted from Pickard J. 1988. A new county classification system. *Appalachia* 21(3):19-24, Summer.

Figure 2-4
Physicians per 100,000 Population, Pickard Classification

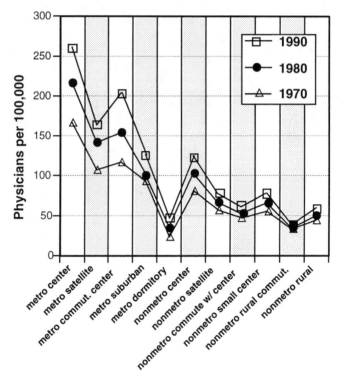

The E/R ratio is the number of workers working in the county divided by the number of workers residing in the county.

Using this classification system illustrates the discontinuity in the rural–urban continuum. Figure 2-4 shows a drop-off in physician supply from the core metropolitan counties toward the suburban and metro fringe counties. However, the supply rises in nonmetro centers and then tapers off again as the nonmetro counties become smaller and more distant.

The Pickard categorization is similar to one used by Clifford, Miller and Stokes (1986) as they explored mortality differences

Figure 2-5

Death Rates per 1,000 Population from All Causes by County of Residence, United States, 1970-1980

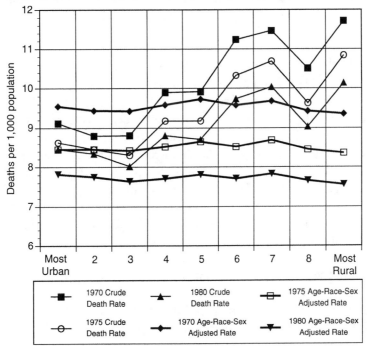

Source: Adapted from Clifford WB, MK Miller, and CS Stokes. 1986. *Rural-urban differences in the United States, 1970-1980.*

within rural types and between rural and urban counties (Figure 2-5). The classification system they used arrayed counties from urban core or fringe metropolitan counties with 1 million or more people to nonmetropolitan, nonadjacent counties with the size of the largest place less than 2,500. That study found higher crude rates of death in rural versus urban areas. These differences were largely explained by the demographics of the county groups. Figure 2-5 compares the crude rates for 1970, 1975, and 1980 with the age-, race-, and sex-adjusted mortality rates for deaths from all causes according to the urban or rural character of the counties.

Figure 2-5 indicates that there are two patterns of change in mortality from more urban to more rural county types. In the crude rates there is an apparent increase in mortality from urban to rural. After adjustment for age, race, and sex, the differences largely disappear.

Mapping Urban and Rural Populations

The distribution of rural versus urban county types will vary according to the system used and the region of the country. The size and number of counties differs markedly between the Eastern and Western regions of the United States. In the series of maps that follows, Figures 2-6 through 2-8, three classification systems are used in choroplethic maps of four states: two with very large urban areas and a mixture of rural types; a mountainous, western state with very large counties; and an upper midwestern state with a single large metropolitan area. The maps show what might be considered smooth gradients from very urban to very rural areas as with Minnesota, or abrupt transitions from urban to very rural in Colorado. The map of Illinois illustrates a more urban corridor between Chicago and St. Louis, with more rural counties peripheral to this axis, while the New York map shows a generally urban state with a few isolated rural counties that appear as "islands" in the choroplethic maps in Figures 2-7 and 2-8.

These classification systems attempt to categorize all counties on some form of rural–urban continuum for general purposes. These classifications result in slightly different clusters of counties that may or may not have relevance to health services distribution and utilization. Health services researchers are sometimes compelled to describe and use their own rural–urban classification system to more closely describe the utilization of services or the distribution of resources.

Examples of the types of classifications discussed above are specific to states or sub-state areas which are the focus of a particular analysis. Figure 2-9, illustrates a customized categorization of the counties in Alabama in order to classify the parts of the

Figure 2-6
Map Examples: AMA County Classification System

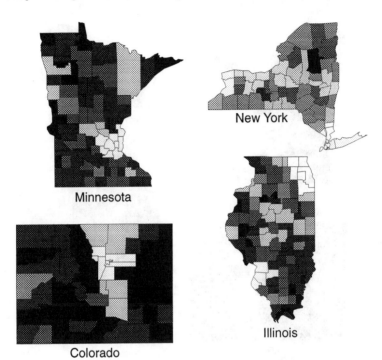

Demographic County Classification

■	1	nonmetropolitan counties; 0 to 9,999
■	2	nonmetropolitan counties; 10,000 to 24,999
▨	3	nonmetropolitan counties; 25,000 to 49,999
▨	4	nonmetropolitan counties; ≥50,000
▨	5	counties considered potential SMSA's
▨	6	counties in SMSA's; 50,000 to 499,999
□	7	counties in SMSA's; 500,000 to 999,999
□	8	counties in SMSA's; 1,000,000 to 4,999,999
□	9	counties in SMSA's; ≥ 5,000,000

Data Source: Area Resource File, ODAM, Bureau of Health Professions, March 1992. Produced by: NC Rural Health Research Program, Cecil G. Sheps Center for Health Services Research, UNC - Chapel Hill.

Figure 2-7

Map Examples: Rural–Urban Continuum Categories

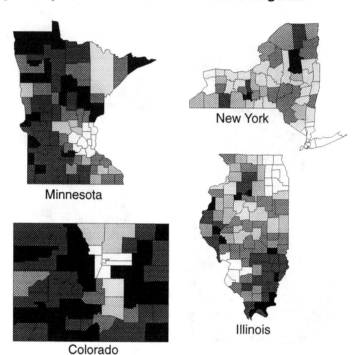

Minnesota

New York

Colorado

Illinois

Continuum Code

☐ 0 large metropolitan core counties
☐ 1 large metropolitan fringe counties
▨ 2 medium metropolitan counties
▨ 3 lesser metropolitan counties
▨ 4 nonmetropolitan, urbanized and adjacent to SMSA
▨ 5 nonmetropolitan, urbanized and nonadjacent to SMSA
▨ 6 nonmetropolitan, less urbanized and adjacent to SMSA
▨ 7 nonmetropolitan, less urbanized and nonadjacent to SMSA
■ 8 nonmetropolitan, thinly populated adjacent to SMSA
■ 9 nonmetropolitan, thinly populated and nonadjacent to SMSA

Data Source: Area Resource File, ODAM, Bureau of Health Professions,
March 1992. Produced by: NC Rural Health Research Program, Cecil G.
Sheps Center for Health Services Research, UNC - Chapel Hill.

Figure 2-8
Map Examples: Pickard Classification System

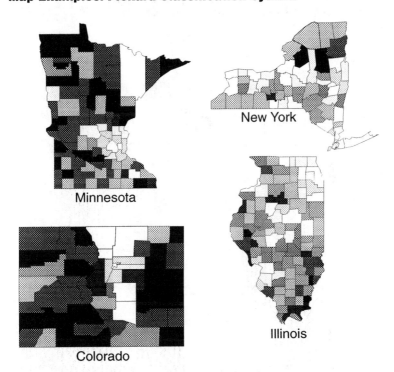

New York

Minnesota

Illinois

Colorado

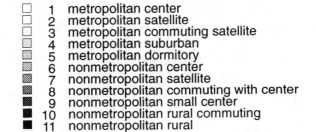

County Type Code

□	1	metropolitan center
□	2	metropolitan satellite
□	3	metropolitan commuting satellite
▨	4	metropolitan suburban
▨	5	metropolitan dormitory
▨	6	nonmetropolitan center
▨	7	nonmetropolitan satellite
▨	8	nonmetropolitan commuting with center
■	9	nonmetropolitan small center
■	10	nonmetropolitan rural commuting
■	11	nonmetropolitan rural

Data Source: Area Resource File, ODAM, Bureau of Health Professions,
March 1992. Produced by: NC Rural Health Research Program, Cecil G.
Sheps Center for Health Services Research, UNC - Chapel Hill.

Figure 2-9

Map Example: Designation of County Types in Alabama for Study of Obstetrical Access

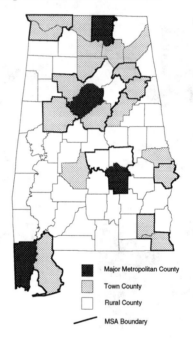

Major Metropolitan County

Town County

Rural County

MSA Boundary

Source: Bronstein JM. 1992. Entrance and exit of obstetrics providers in rural Alabama. *Journal of Rural Health* 8(2):114-120.

state with regard to changes in the supply of obstetrical providers (Bronstein, 1992). The principal criteria for categorization were population and metropolitan designation but the system produced five classes of county: major metropolitan county, metropolitan "town," metropolitan rural, town, and rural county. The utility of the map depended on how well it reflected the distribution of resources in Alabama.

New York has developed its own classification of the rural–urban continuum (Figure 2-10) to reflect the range of conditions in that state (New York State Legislative Commission on Rural Resources, 1990). The geography of New York identifies

Figure 2-10
Classification of New York State Counties

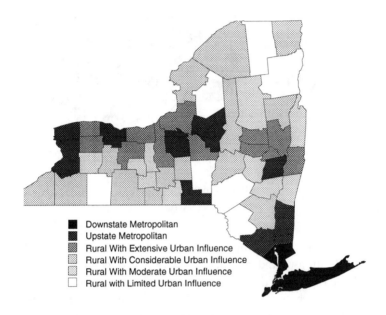

Source: New York State Legislative Commission on Rural Resources, 1990.

certain types of rural and urban counties and the special situation, geographically and in the distribution of resources, of the New York City metropolitan area. The system identifies six categories: Rural with Limited Urban Influence, Rural with Moderate Urban Influence, Rural with Considerable Urban Influence, Rural with Extensive Urban Influence, Upstate Metropolitan, and Downstate Metropolitan.

A final map example included (Figure 2-11) was developed to reflect the distribution of cancer care resources in North Carolina for a study of the relationship of rurality to stage at diagnosis for cancer care patients (Monroe, Aldrich, Ricketts & Cooper, 1992). The counties that had high levels of cancer care, as measured by the number of medical oncologists, were both metropolitan and

Figure 2-11
County Classification by Availability of Cancer Care

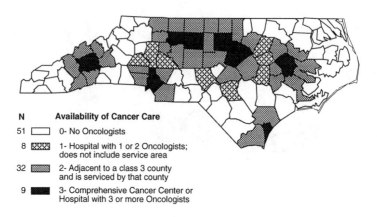

nonmetropolitan. A simple classification was developed based on OMB definitions and included a county with a medical school and a major oncology department as rural and one county with no hospital as urban. This classification system was then modified to classify the counties as "central" with regard to oncology resources or "peripheral." The intention was originally to draw conclusions concerning rurality and cancer care but the distribution of resources meant that comparisons had to be made within categories of rural and urban. The urban counties with no oncologists were compared to rural counties with no oncologists to try to identify a rural effect.

The Rural–Urban Continuum and Health Services Research

Many studies in health services as well as clinical research seek to determine small area differences in use of services, the performance of organizations, or outcomes of care. The determination of a measure of rurality or urbanity for use in studies that examine geographic differences depends upon the research questions being addressed. If the study is one that examines the ability of persons to keep follow-up appointments for sexually transmitted disease treatment, then the rural orientation of the individuals should be measured along with their perceptions of the difficulty of traveling to the clinic or caregiver. The first measure is one of rurality for the individual patient or user, the second is a spatial measure not necessarily tied to rural or urban location.

If a study is meant to determine the differences in the financial performance of hospitals under various Health Care Financing Administration payment systems based on geography, the determination of rural has been made by the federal agency and rurality is whatever the agency says it is. If, however, the analyst is concerned with varying definitions of rural that are meant to capture the relative effect of isolation and distance from suppliers or the effects of labor markets on hospital costs, then the definition of rural would be spatial and would depend upon distance measures, prevailing labor rates within jurisdictions or geographically-defined areas, and the local costs of transportation. In this case the definition of rural would be specific to hospital costs and would deviate from a more general concept of rurality.

The desire to identify a common and consistent definition and scale of rurality has caused consternation among many researchers and analysts as they have tried to apply general policy prescriptions meant to benefit "rural" people through the specifics of a financing or service program. This consternation would not lead to confusion or programmatic delay if policy makers and analysts alike recognized that rural is not a precise concept. Rather, policy makers, and, more directly, those who write regulations, should recognize that there are many different available measures of rurality that can be used more or less appropriately in assigning areas or people to one or more classes for benefits or targeted programs.

Policy makers in the political arena attempt to create coalitions that bring many different kinds of "rural" people under one program or into a benefit arrangement. This tendency is the source of much of the problem in trying to meet the intentions of legislation meant to benefit "rural" communities and people.

▷ P O I N T
▷ OF DEPARTURE

Population Density and Research

Diana N. Osborne and Lucy A. Savitz

Population Density Defined

There exist various typologies for characterizing an area of land, usually a county, in terms of its population concentration; examples of classification schemas are urban versus rural, or metropolitan versus nonmetropolitan. These classifications are in turn used to make decisions about placement of health care facilities and providers and in planning for potential health infrastructure needs. Population density, a measure of population concentration, is one component of the basis for rural/urban classifications, and is usually used in conjunction with population size, adjacency to metropolitan areas, and urbanization (Hewitt, 1992). In this Point of Departure we focus on population density, its use in health services research, and a specific instance of very low population density: frontier counties.

Computation

Population density can be defined as the number of people per unit area in a society, region, or country, and is a measure of the intensity of settlement of a region (Austin et al., 1987). Population density is determined by dividing the resident population of a geographic unit by the land area it occupies, usually expressed in the US as square miles. In

1990, two percent of the US population was living in counties with ten or fewer persons per square mile. In the United States as of 1990, population density ranged from .15 persons per square mile in Loving County, Texas to 67,613 persons per square mile in New York County, New York (Area Resource File, 1992).

Interpretation

Population density is limited as a descriptor in that it does not give any indication of how population is distributed within the area being examined. For example a county that is large in area, as is common in the western United States, may contain a densely urbanized area as well as large areas that are sparsely populated. Population density measured at the county level would tend to mask these extremes.

Use in Health Services Research

The determination of appropriate levels of health care services available in a given region is generally based on the size of the service area and the number of individuals it is anticipated will be using the services. Although there are many variables involved in who will obtain what health services in what location, clearly size of service area and the population it contains are inextricably related. A facility serving a square mile in a city with a population density of greater than 10,000 people will have different priorities and needs in terms of staffing and services provided than will a facility serving a large western county with a population density of six to ten persons per square mile. This point becomes apparent when viewing a map of California counties (Figure 2-12). Different service levels are or are not sustainable at differing population densities. Determining the most efficient means of making available an appropriate level of care in a specific location requires closer examination to discern where the most and least densely populated areas are located within the area of study.

Figure 2-12
Population Density by County, California, 1986

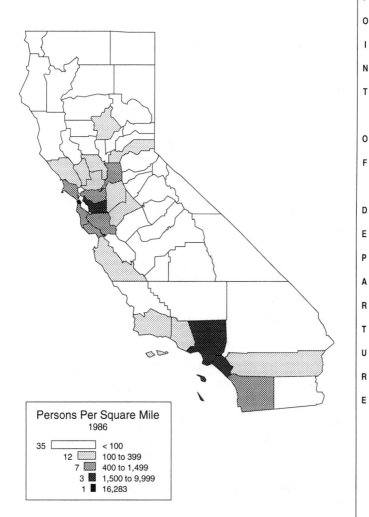

Persons Per Square Mile
1986

35	< 100
12	100 to 399
7	400 to 1,499
3	1,500 to 9,999
1	16,283

Data Source: Strategic Mapping, Inc.

Frontier Areas, A Special Case

In response to ongoing concerns that the health care needs of rural areas were not being adequately met, various classification systems have been developed. One of these, the frontier county designation, is an offshoot of the "frontier" concept that has become a part of the American collective consciousness (Popper, 1986). Some schools of thought would say there is no longer any "frontier" area in the US, and, in fact, this would not be a new argument. As a result of the 1890 decennial census, the Census Superintendent stated that " 'Up to and including 1880 the country had a frontier of settlement, but at present the unsettled area has been so broken into by isolated bodies of settlement that there can hardly be said to be a frontier line. In the discussion of its extent, its westward movement, etc., it can not, therefore, any longer have a place in the census reports' " (No more frontier?, 1993). An early look at the 1990 Census, however, showed that there remain 150 counties in the US that still meet the old census definition of frontier land—fewer than two persons per square mile. All of these counties are west of the 98th meridian, which is the 19th century "frontier line."

Definition

In modern day discussions of health care provision, "frontier" is applied at the county level, and can denote from six to ten persons per square mile; in most cases frontier is defined as six or fewer persons per square mile. Demographer Frank Popper found that as late as 1984, using a definition of six or fewer persons per square mile, there were 394 counties, constituting 45% of the US land area, that would meet the standard (Elison, 1986). Figure 2-13 depicts 1990 "frontier" counties at various population levels.

Relationship to Rural

Interest in frontier areas picked up around 1985. At this time rural providers, public health planning staff, and US

Figure 2-13   Frontier Counties, 1990, by Nonmetropolitan County

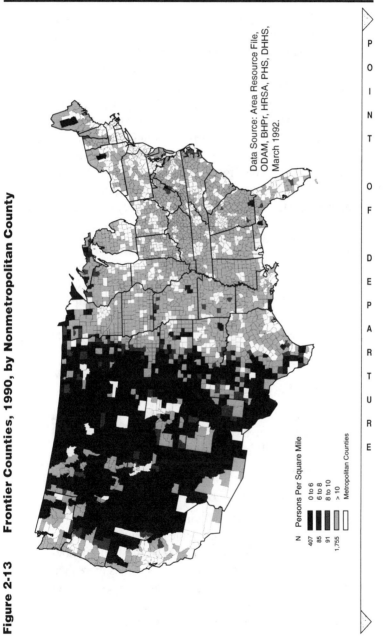

Data Source: Area Resource File,
ODAM, BHPr, HRSA, PHS, DHHS,
March 1992.

Persons Per Square Mile

407   0 to 6
85   6 to 8
91   8 to 10
1,755 > 10
      Metropolitan Counties

POINT OF DEPARTURE

Department of Health and Human Services staff agreed that frontier areas constituted a unique setting in terms of service delivery and should accordingly be considered under different criteria than those used for urban or rural service areas (Elison, 1986). A Frontier Health Care Task Force was convened, under sponsorship of HHS Regions VII and VIII, to look at health issues as they applied to frontier areas and try to identify those characteristics distinguishing urban, rural and frontier settings in terms of access to health care services. The work of this task force, in conjunction with the National Rural Health Association, led to modified guidelines for the approval of federal assistance to community health centers in frontier areas. Their guidelines included these alternative definitions (Elison, 1986):

> Service Area: a rational area in the frontier will have at least 500 residents within a 25-mile radius of the health service delivery site or within a logical trade area. Most areas will have between 500-3,000 residents and cover large geographic areas.

> Population Density: the service area will have six or fewer persons per square mile.

> Distance: the service area will be such that the distance from the primary care site to the next level of care will be more than 45 miles and/or 60 minutes.

Related Health Service Delivery Issues

For frontier areas, the primary service delivery issue is how best to overcome geographic distance and spatial isolation (Cordes, 1989). In many large western counties the nearest health care facility, a rural hospital, is more than 100 miles away. After receiving initial emergency treatment there, a patient may be referred to a tertiary care center another 100-200 miles away. In many instances, distances of this length can cause significant problems of access, such as for a pregnant woman requiring a series of prenatal visits and eventually delivery. In general, "low population density means that the scale of operation of the medical system in rural areas will be noticeably smaller and different than in urban areas. Indeed, ... it is this characteristic that often leads to fundamental and intrinsic differences in the way health services are delivered, including the use of airborne ambulances, telecommunication linkages between remote outposts and secondary care centers, and satellite care centers staffed with physician assistants and nurse practitioners" (Study of models, 1992).

Distance to care must be considered in terms of travel time required, as well as availability of transportation. Accordingly, many believe that the unique delivery problems of frontier areas require solutions different from those that may be successful in urban or rural areas.

Low population density can affect health care needs as well as delivery. Some research suggests that high rates of alcohol abuse and suicide in very rural areas may be related to the large physical distances separating people which "make social networking and the formation of psychological support groups difficult to establish and maintain" (Study of models, 1992).

Population density has statistical implications as well. A yearly infant mortality rate has very limited meaning in a rural location where there are only a few births per year. Because of low volume, facilities located in these sparsely populated areas may not be able to absorb catastrophic financial losses for even a single incident of high-cost uncompensated care. While it may not be feasible to keep all rural hospitals open with a full spectrum of care available, provisions must be made such that primary care and emergency services remain accessible. The effect of population size on the development of rural medical services is depicted in Figure 2-14. This chart

POINT OF DEPARTURE

Figure 2-14
Effect of Population Size on Development of Rural Medical Services

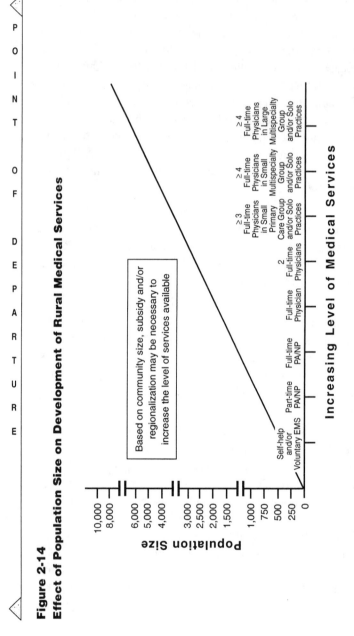

Source: Adapted from Baldwin DC, and B Rowley. 1990. Alternative models for the delivery of rural health care: A case study of a western frontier state. *Journal of Rural Health* 6(3):256-272.

depicts, from a financial perspective, the level of care sustainable without some amount of subsidization or an attempt to create a formal or informal regional network of services.

Identifying what is the most efficient type of health care facility in these areas, how to procure staff for that facility, and how to induce those staff to stay are enduring problems for rural areas, and especially frontier areas, where small centers of population are separated by large distances. Many frontier areas will require a financial subsidy to be able to support even a single physician, and in some settings nurse practitioners, physician assistants and/or certified nurse midwives may be more appropriate providers of care. In a study in Nevada looking at alternative care settings, the authors noted that the models that showed promise usually "developed indigenously on the basis of what seems to work locally, rather than according to any ideal model or concept of rural health care" (Baldwin & Rowley, 1990). Policy makers attempting to tackle the problem of providing an adequate level of health services to frontier populations may find it useful to develop more flexible approaches that incorporate multiple and innovative configurations of facilities and providers.

POINT OF DEPARTURE

Chapter 3

Changes and Measures in the Crucial Dimension of Population

Point of Departure:
Data Sources for Health Services Research

Any study of the geographic pattern, or spatial distribution, of fertility and mortality has to start with the distribution of the population itself and all the varied elements that compose it. Next, there is a need to demographically differentiate types of areas, as the need for health services is related to the age and gender of the population as well as economic and ethnic factors. The changes occurring in migration, fertility and mortality have different spatial distributions, and in turn affect the distribution of the elements of population, projections of population, and estimates of future needs for health services.

Shifts in population distribution and related changes in health care utilization within an area illustrate the need for planning and adaptability. One extreme example of the need to plan and adapt would be changes in the population and health care needs in Florida. That state has heavy in-migration from foreign countries, by young adults from other states drawn by employment opportunities, and by retirees seeking a favorable climate. Morbidity and mortality, fertility, and mobility in Florida will change as a result of the migration, and these patterns must be considered before projections of health resource need are completed. This concern with the composition, distribution, and dynamics of population is part of the content of population geography. In this chapter, the dynamics of fertility, mortality, and migration are discussed and a variety of measurements and techniques from population geography are introduced and used to describe and analyze population in ways relevant to health conditions and service delivery.

Population Composition

The *elements of population* include characteristics such as age, gender, race, ethnicity, education, religion, occupation, and dietary preference. While such characteristics have an impact on disease ecology, the effect of age is overwhelming. In this section, we will consider age structure and its impact on the dynamics of population: fertility, mortality, and mobility.

Crude birth rates for a population are of minimal use for planning or analysis since they are calculated as:

Crude Birth Rate =

$$\frac{\text{\# of Live Births During a Calendar Year}}{\text{Total, Mid-Year Population}} \times 1{,}000$$

This crude rate may conceal changes in fertility behavior by obscuring the contribution being made by different groups of childbearing-age women as well as the age mix of the population. In general, crude birth rates are used to indicate the impact of fertility on population growth. For this reason, *total fertility rates*, which are based on age-specific rates (either single year or often 5-year age ranges), make better summary measures for population dynamics. Both general and total fertility rate measures relate the number of births to the population at risk (women between the ages of 15 and 44) whereby the general and total fertility rates are calculated as follows:

General Fertility Rate =

$$\frac{\text{\# of Live Births to All Women in a Calendar Year}}{\substack{\text{Mid-Year Population of Women} \\ \text{15-44 Years of Age}}} \quad \text{x } 1{,}000$$

Total Fertility Rate =

The sum of age-specific birth rates of women at each age group (e.g., 10-14 through 45-49). When multi-year age groups are used, the sum is accordingly multiplied (five-year age groups are multiplied by 5).

Age-Specific Birth Rate =

$$\frac{\substack{\text{\# of Live Births to Women in a} \\ \text{Specific Age Group During a Calendar Year}}}{\substack{\text{Mid-Year Population of Women} \\ \text{in the Same Age Group}}} \quad \text{x } 1{,}000$$

Age-specific birth rates are commonly relied upon to evaluate population growth. Cefalo and Gay (1988) provide a thorough discussion of the differences in these rates.

Figure 3-1 illustrates different fertility behavior by age and race of American women using age-specific birth rates (US National Center for Health Statistics, 1991). With more than four million births per year in 1990, the highest since 1963, the United States has been having a baby boomlet. After increasing three percent a year from 1988 to 1989 to 1990, however, births started to fall two percent a year in 1991 and the trend has continued (US NCHS, 1992). This results from the fact that the larger part of the population born in the 1950's, the "baby boom" age cohort, has passed through their childbearing years; even without changes in

Figure 3-1
US Fertility Behavior by Age and Race, 1989

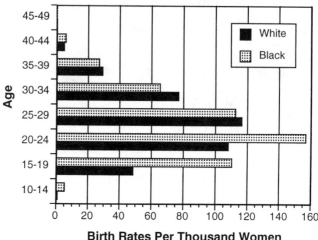

Birth Rates Per Thousand Women

fertility behavior, the smaller numbers of women in succeeding age cohorts will have fewer births. The crude birth rate for 1990 was 16.7 per 1,000 women, 16.2 for 1991, and 15.8 for December 1991 alone. Age-specific birth rates for women between 1988 and 1990 increased to the highest rates in 15 years for teenagers and for women 35-44 years of age. Births to women aged 40-44 totaled 44,401 in 1989, compared to 22,627 in 1978 (US NCHS, 1991), reflecting the continued trend of postponed childbearing and increased female participation in the labor force (Morrill, 1993). In 1989, the general fertility rate for white women was 66.0 live births per 1,000 women aged 15-44, and for black women it was 85.8. Despite some increase in births for each age category, the total fertility rate was still below replacement reproduction as it has been since 1972.

Because fertility behavior is so closely related to age, both the mobility of women and the local female population's age structure will have strong impacts on demand for obstetrical and gynecological services or facilities. These differ between rural and urban areas as well as among subregions of a state.

The impact of age structure on causes of *mortality* and *morbidity* is even more important since these analyses include a full century of experience and are not based solely on females of childbearing age. [The mortality and morbidity associations at different stages of the life cycle are described more fully elsewhere (Meade, 1992).] Figures 3-2 through 3-5 illustrate some of the structural variation by age. The age structure of total mortality conforms to the expected image of increase with age (Figure 3-2). Death from a degenerative disease like diabetes rapidly picks up after age 54 (Figure 3-3). AIDS (Figure 3-4) kills infants, teens, and young adults, but as a cause of death affects mostly young and middle-aged adults from 25 to 54. Finally, motor vehicle accidents kill young adults at the highest rate, although the motor vehicle is a great equalizer, killing younger children, middle-aged persons, and senior citizens at similar rates (Figure 3-5). Preventive practices and health education vary from place to place (spatially) and over time (temporally), of course, but changes in age structure would easily be the dominant factor in changes in demand for various types of facilities or specialists. Eliminating the statistical confounding introduced by variance in age structure among populations is a prerequisite to virtually all analyses of cause of death, so research almost routinely controls for age by arithmetic adjustments (as described in the Point of Departure accompanying Chapter 8). It should be noted that there are different purposes for standardization of rates that involve the comparison of populations, usually for disease rates. However, unadjusted incidence and prevalence rates are used for the provision of health care and targeting program interventions for specific populations.

The dynamic of population *mobility* is probably the most underestimated factor in age structure and medical need. Mobility is the umbrella term subsuming microscale circulation as well as macroscale migration. Mobility is of primary importance in studies of exposure to hazards and problems of analyzing disease etiology. Population *migration*, which involves change of residence (across a political boundary such as a county), is of primary importance in determining the age structure and other elements of population

Figure 3-2
North Carolina Mortality by Age, 1990

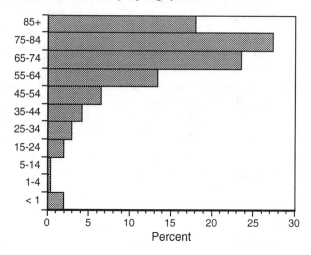

Figure 3-3
North Carolina Mortality by Age for Diabetes Mellitus, 1990

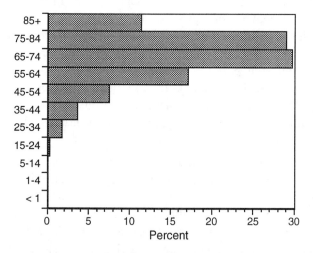

Data Source: North Carolina Center for Health and Environmental Statistics, 1991.
Produced by: NC Rural Health Research Program, Cecil G. Sheps Center for Health
Services Research, UNC - Chapel Hill.

Figure 3-4
North Carolina Mortality by Age for AIDS, 1990

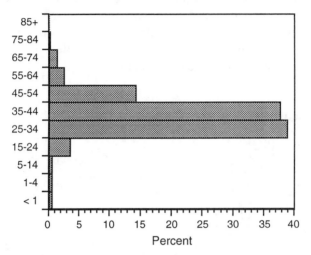

Figure 3-5
North Carolina Mortality by Age for Motor Vehicle Accidents, 1990

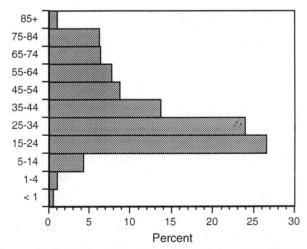

Data Source: North Carolina Center for Health and Environmental Statistics, 1991. Produced by: NC Rural Health Research Program, Cecil G. Sheps Center for Health Services Research, UNC - Chapel Hill.

composition. The US Bureau of the Census uses the term mobility in an intermediate sense, to mean moving residence. Such a move may be from one apartment to another in the same building, or it may be to a different school district within the same county or city, or it may be to a different country. Some of the different patterns of US population mobility are illustrated in Figure 3-6.

Figure 3-6
US Population Mobility, 1989-90

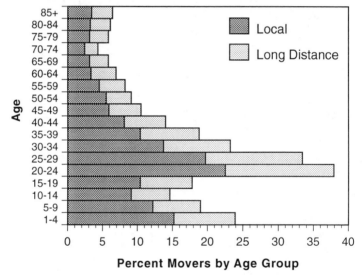

Percent Movers by Age Group

Source: Data from Table F, Selected Characteristics of Persons, by Mobility Status and Type of Move: 1989-90. Bureau of the Census, US Department of Commerce.

The importance of change of life stage (marriage, first job, first child, retirement, etc.) as a reason to move is well known. It is reflected in Figure 3-6 in the mobility of small children (more local) and young adults. Retirement migration gets a lot of attention, primarily because its impact is so spatially focused. As the figure illustrates, mobility of those over 60 is the lowest. It increases slightly at the oldest ages as people move to institutional care or to reside with their children. Roughly 18 percent of the US population moved from 1989-1990 (down from over 20 percent in the 1950's and 1960's), but more than half of the moves were local ones within the same county. Analysis of data from the US Bureau of the Census (1991) suggests obvious mobility discrepancies among specific subgroups. Whether for jobs, education, or marriage, those in their twenties move at the highest rates, but as they move up the age structure and have teenagers in secondary school, this group becomes tied down. Of non-farm households, 22.1 percent moved; conversely, only 15.1 percent of farm households moved. Mobility differences by race were noted such that 17.3 percent of whites, 20.2 percent of blacks, and 25.1 percent of Hispanics moved. Similarly, differences in mobility associated with education were observed where for those over 25 years of age: 11.2 percent with eight or fewer years of education, 14.6 percent with a high school education, and 17.9 percent of those with four years of college moved. Home ownership was related to a relatively lower level of mobility with 9.2 percent of homeowners moving, compared with 35.7 percent of renters. The impact of these moves, as related to need for health services, can be simply depicted in population pyramids.

Population pyramids offer a snapshot of what a certain population's age structure is like at a given time. A population pyramid is basically a kind of bar graph in which males are represented on the left side of a vertical line and females on the right (by convention). The impact of various age-specific rates of mortality, fertility, and mobility can then be visualized. (Similarly, the simplest kind of population projection is to look at the pyramid and mentally move the bars up five or ten years, allowing for attrition at the top.) The question is then asked sequentially for each year, or for five-year increments, "What percentage of the population is male and aged less than one? Female? What percentage is male and aged one? Female and aged one? ... Male and aged 50?" and so on; the appropriate percentage is marked off on a piece of graph paper (or, of course, with a more elaborate computerized spread sheet and graphic system). Individual years can be used, but usually five-year categories are sufficient. The bars can be subdivided further by race, income, or other relevant category. Pyramids can also be constructed using absolute numbers rather than percentages; the question then becomes, "How many people are female and aged over 90?" This type of pyramid is effective and even easier to construct since it requires no calculations, but it is difficult to compare the pyramids of large and small populations with each other so percentages are more useful for purposes of comparison.

The term "pyramid" is taken from the shape representing the distribution for populations which are at an early phase along the demographic or epidemiologic transition. In any population, major causes of death are related to levels of economic and institutional development. The generalizations associated with this model are based on the US and European experiences and may not be relevant for the Third World. Nevertheless, the spectrum of development ranges from low levels, which are characterized by high birth and death rates and relatively low life expectancies (most people die of infectious diseases and epidemics), to higher levels of development at the end of the demographic transition, which are characterized by declining birth and death rates with much greater life expectancies at birth (degenerative diseases are the major causes of death). Therefore, the classic pyramid in effect reflects the fact that populations at early phases of the demographic transition experience high birth and mortality rates; connecting the center point of all the bars creates a broad-based pyramid. For countries late in the demographic transition, with low fertility, mortality, and growth, a rectangle is often a more accurate description of the resulting shape.

Figures 3-7 and 3-8 illustrate the population pyramids of two rural counties in the United States for 1990. Comparing the age-specific graphs of Figures 3-1 and 3-2 with the pyramids will make the importance of different health problems and related service demand among the counties more evident. The role of mobility in creating the structures is discussed later.

Figure 3-7
Population Pyramid: Sweetwater County, Wyoming, 1990

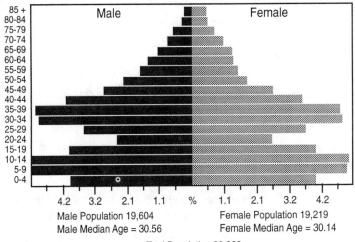

Male Population 19,604
Male Median Age = 30.56

Female Population 19,219
Female Median Age = 30.14

Total Population 38,823
Median Age = 30.35

Figure 3-8
Population Pyramid: Marion County, Florida, 1990

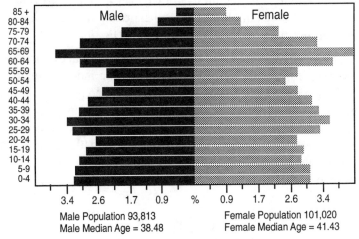

Male Population 93,813
Male Median Age = 38.48

Female Population 101,020
Female Median Age = 41.43

Total Population 194,833
Median Age = 39.96

Techniques Used to Analyze Population Distribution

Several techniques for measuring and comparing distributions of populations at risk or in need have been developed and are useful at a variety of scales. One of the first steps in assessing existing services and projecting future need is to measure and understand the current distribution of subsets of the population at particular risk or in need of various services. In this section, we describe the Lorenz curve, location quotients, demographic base maps, and population potential as possible tools for examining population.

Measures of population distribution are sometimes depicted with aspatial graphic solutions, or "divergency graphs," which show the differences between distributions. Tri-factor graphs which measure characteristics of the population (usually as percentages of selected categories) against three axes are now seldom used because they are difficult to read and interpret. Far more popular are *Lorenz curves*, which measure accumulated percentages of two distributions along their respective axes. Divergence from the "equal" distribution can be compared among populations by assessing the distance from the ideal diagonal line. (A general example of this is provided as Figure 4-3 in Chapter 4, *Access to Health Services*, and an example of the application of this technique is presented in Chapter 5, *Health Professions Distribution.*)

The *location quotient* (LQ) is a measure of spatial distribution convenient for a wide range of topics. It is an index of relative distribution calculated as a proportion of proportions; the resulting location quotients are easily sketched out on a work map. LQs are relevant when the spatial pattern, not statistical correlation of variables, is of interest. This measure can be especially useful when detailed data for current age adjustment and fine categories for rates are not available. The basic formula is:

$$\frac{A_i/\sum A_i}{T_i/\sum T_i} \quad \text{where:}$$

A is the value for the sub-category;

T the value of the total, or whole category; and

i each areal unit being mapped.

The LQ equals the proportion of a variable or resource in an area divided by the proportion of that resource or variable in the aggregate. Figure 3-9 shows LQs mapped for the three relative distributions for motor vehicle accidents, black population, and infant deaths for the eleven-county Health Service Area IV in North Carolina.

Calculation of LQs is demonstrated as:

$$\frac{\% \text{ of total regional activity in area i}}{\% \text{ of total base activity in area i}}$$

The selection of the base or standard distribution used in the denominator is subjective but should take on some logical meaning. Usually, if the activities are part of an aggregate, then the aggregate distribution is used to estimate the base. However, it is also possible to use area populations or actual land area as the standard of comparison (e.g., percent of core physicians divided by the percent of total physicians).

As a ratio of two percentages, the LQ is dimensionless, ranging from 0 to infinity and can be interpreted as follows:

$LQ_i > 1$ relative concentration of the activity in area i compared to the region as a whole.

$LQ_i < 1$ area i has less of a share of the activity in accordance with its share of the base.

$LQ_i = 1$ area i has a share of activity in accordance with the base.

Spatial patterns of inequality can be revealed by mapping these LQs. A major disadvantage is that a single number is calculated for

Figure 3-9 **Mapping of Locational Quotients for North Carolina Health Service Area IV**

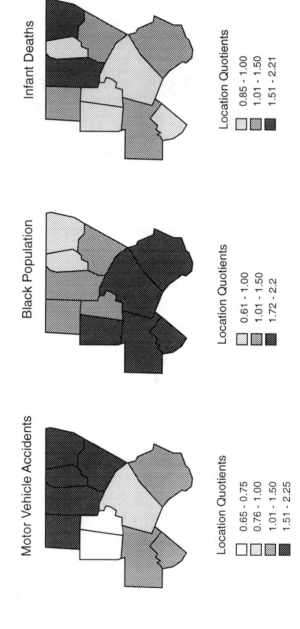

Data Source: NC CHES, 1991.
Produced by: NC Rural Health Research Program, Cecil G. Sheps Center for Health Services Research, UNC - Chapel Hill.

each area being considered. Thus, a large number of areas (e.g., Census tracts in major urban areas) yield a large number of LQs, resulting in an inefficient form of summary, even when mapped. LQs are simple to calculate and easily understood and therefore can be quite useful in the early, exploratory stages of research. It should be cautioned that the observed fact that a subarea has more or less of a proportionate share of a larger area's activity is not particularly informative. Careful interpretation of results and thoughtful development of policy resulting from these observations are recommended. The use of LQs is also discussed in Chapter 5, *Health Professions Distribution*.

Table 3-1 illustrates the calculation of location quotients for the distribution of the black population for the 11 counties of Health Service Area IV. In this case, total population is the base. First, the proportion of total county population relative to that of the State is determined. Similarly, the proportion of the black population relative to the total black population for the State is calculated. The county-specific proportion of black population is divided by the county-specific proportion of total population to arrive at the LQ for each county.

Demographic base maps (DBM) eliminate the distortion of spatial pattern created by representing population events on an areal base. For example, the prevalence of AIDS mapped at the state level might indicate a statewide problem in Colorado, while the majority of that state's population is virtually confined to the area east of the Rockies between Boulder and Pueblo with the exception of a few small, isolated towns across the state. In a DBM, the size of a unit is proportional to the number of people it contains. In the standard map of the United States, the giant, arid, and mountainous states of the West occupy half the country such that any high rate mapped upon them becomes dramatically important in a visual sense. On a DBM reflecting any population attribute, those states are significantly reduced, and it is the rates mapped upon densely populated states like California, Florida, and New York that dominate the visual message. These maps can be constructed by race, age,

Table 3-1
Work Table for Location Quotients

County	Total Population	Total Proportion	Black Population	Black Proportion	LQs
Johnston	81,306	0.0796	14,389	0.0538	0.68
Durham	181,835	0.1780	67,654	0.2530	1.42
Chatham	38,759	0.0379	8,843	0.0331	0.87
Lee	41,374	0.0405	9,401	0.0351	0.87
Wake	423,380	0.4144	88,057	0.3292	0.79
Orange	93,851	0.0919	14,893	0.0557	0.61
Franklin	36,414	0.0356	12,843	0.0480	1.35
Warren	17,265	0.0169	9,847	0.0368	2.18
Vance	38,892	0.0381	17,512	0.0655	1.72
Granville	38,345	0.0375	14,909	0.0557	1.49
Person	30,180	0.0295	9,106	0.0340	1.15
Total	1,021,601	1.0000	267,454	1.0000	

gender, or any other subgroup of the population for which numbers are available. Thus, a program concerned with preschool vaccination, or meals for the elderly, or family planning for teenagers could map their service rates of interest upon a base map of the targeted population. Shading of subunits could be used to illustrate the proportion living alone or in poverty. The map depicts the relative as well as absolute number of cases needing or getting services.

Figure 3-10 shows the construction of a DBM. To create a DBM, use a sheet of graph paper, and subjectively determine the number of people in the target population that should be represented by one square. Starting with the largest unit, block off the appropriate number of squares, proceeding outward. For a DBM to be

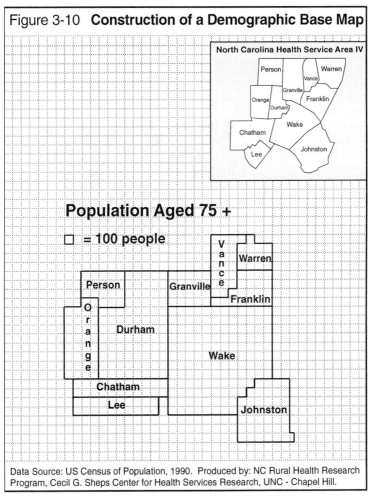

Figure 3-10   **Construction of a Demographic Base Map**

Data Source: US Census of Population, 1990. Produced by: NC Rural Health Research Program, Cecil G. Sheps Center for Health Services Research, UNC - Chapel Hill.

comprehensible, two things must be maintained: contiguity of spatial units, and direction. In other words, two counties that do or do not touch (are or are not contiguous) should be so depicted. Counties that are east/west of each other cannot be drawn north/ south or no one will recognize them. Maintaining the contiguity and direction of areal units—while their size is many times altered by representation of population—can be a challenge and a work of art.

Figure 3-11
Areal Base Map
Health Service Area IV, North Carolina

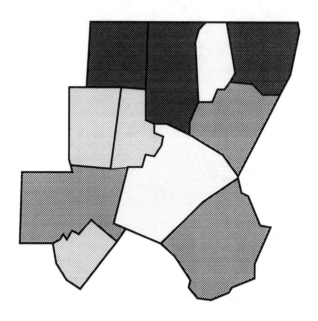

Infant Mortality
per 1,000

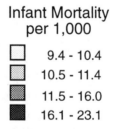

9.4 - 10.4
10.5 - 11.4
11.5 - 16.0
16.1 - 23.1

Data Source: NC CHES, Leading Causes of Mortality, NC Vital Statistics 1989, vol. 2.
Produced by: NC Rural Health Research Program, Cecil G. Sheps Center for Health
Services Research, UNC - Chapel Hill.

Figure 3-12
Demographic Base Map
Health Service Area IV, North Carolina

Area Proportional to Number of People

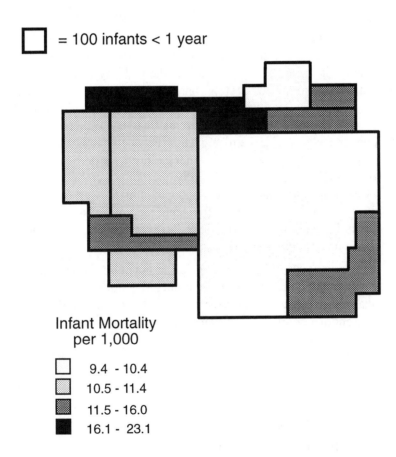

☐ = 100 infants < 1 year

Infant Mortality
per 1,000

☐ 9.4 - 10.4
▦ 10.5 - 11.4
▨ 11.5 - 16.0
■ 16.1 - 23.1

Data Source: NC CHES, Leading Causes of Mortality, NC Vital Statistics 1989, vol. 2.
Produced by: NC Rural Health Research Program, Cecil G. Sheps Center for Health
Services Research, UNC - Chapel Hill.

The human eye and a good eraser are still at times more useful than a computer algorithm. Interpretation is greatly aided by including the standard map as a reference until users become accustomed to the transformation.

Figures 3-11 and 3-12 present the areal and demographic base maps for infant mortality in Health Service Area IV. Notice the change between the standard map and the DBM in the visual communication of the problem of high rates for the region.

Population potential is a measure of distribution that describes the nearness or accessibility of people to a certain point or place. For instance, it could be used to evaluate the viability of a particular medical specialty or service (e.g., oncology, MRI) in locating health care resources. It is closely related to the *gravity model* (described in the Point of Departure accompanying Chapter 7), but rather than being concerned with the relationships between pairs of points, it measures the influence of all other points to a particular one. Population potential was originally part of a set of measures developed to study the "physics" of population (Stewart & Warntz, 1958). The others, statistical "moments" and modes analogous to standard deviations of distributions, have seen little use, but population potential has a wide range of applications.

The general formula for population potential represented by "I", and its interaction (population potential) for each point i, is equal to the population of the point divided by the distance between it and another point summed over all the points measured such that:

$$I_i = \sum_{j=1}^{n} \frac{P_j}{D_{ij}} \quad \text{where:}$$

j is not equal to i;

P is the population of point j;

D_{ij} is the distance between points i and j; and

n is the number of points in the system.

Table 3-2 shows the work table necessary to calculate population potential for the 11 counties of Health Service Area IV given total population; Table 3-3 gives the distances required for the calculations.

Table 3-2
Work Table for Population Potential

County	Total Population	Total Potential
Johnston	81,306	502
Durham	181,835	608
Chatham	38,759	403
Lee	41,374	395
Wake	423,380	687
Orange	93,851	564
Franklin	36,414	411
Warren	17,265	311
Vance	38,892	366
Granville	38,345	481
Person	30,180	394
Total	1,021,601	N/A

Table 3-3
Distances for Calculating Population Potential

County	J	D	C	L	W	O	F	W	V	G	P
Johnston	1.00										
Durham	3.50	1.00									
Chatham	3.95	2.60	1.00								
Lee	3.75	3.40	1.20	1.00							
Wake	1.50	2.10	2.40	2.40	1.00						
Orange	4.00	1.00	1.85	2.90	2.4	1.00					
Franklin	2.90	2.50	4.85	4.90	2.65	3.50	1.00				
Warren	4.45	3.40	5.85	6.30	4.1	4.40	1.55	1.00			
Vance	4.30	2.65	5.20	5.80	3.7	3.60	1.50	0.9	1.00		
Granville	3.75	1.40	3.90	4.60	2.8	2.35	1.6	2.1	1.3	1.00	
Person	5.00	1.65	3.75	4.80	3.70	2.00	3.25	3.42	2.6	1.5	1.00

For the population potential between Durham and Johnston counties, we would have:

181,835/3.5 + 181,835/1 + 181,835/2.6 + 181,835/3.4

+ 181,835/2.1 + 181,835/1 + 181,835/1 + 181,835/2.5

+ 181,835/3.4 + 181,835/2.65 + 181,835/1.4 + 181,835/1.65

= **608**

The potential numbers are large so they are expressed as thousands to make mappable numbers. These values are then, as seen in Figure 3-13, graphically presented as isolines, connecting points of equal population potential that are interpolated to create a mapped surface of accessibility. Such maps are useful for predicting the directional movement of epidemics, which move toward places of greatest accessibility, as well as in optimizing service location.

Population potential is a flexible and versatile measure of distribution, but one must be aware of pitfalls in calculating it for particular purposes. The greatest of these pitfalls results from complications of scale. On one hand, potential is a relative measure so it would seem that it would matter little whether one used miles on the ground or inches measured on a map—locations would still be relatively higher or lower to each other in potential. Since populations are being divided by the distances, the relative effect of distance in differentiating accessibility can vary greatly if small populations are divided by millions of millimeters or dozens of miles. This is much less problematic for larger populations, but when in doubt, use real-world measures. Scale also becomes an issue when the "point" from which distance is measured has area. For example, distances in Figure 3-13 are calculated from the geometric center point in counties—essentially putting population at a point without area or dimension. If towns or other specific points are considered to be actually central to population location, the central point for measuring could be located there so long as all units were treated consistently. If one were to measure potential among several large buildings close together (e.g., high-rise condo-

Figure 3-13

Population Potential Maps
Health Service Area IV, North Carolina

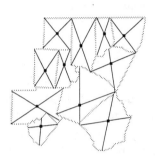

Location of a Geometric Center
for Calculation of Distance

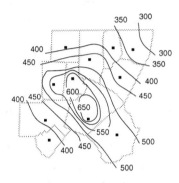

Population Potential (000)
Total Population

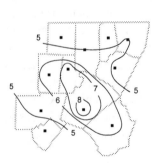

Population Potential (000)
Infants Aged > 1

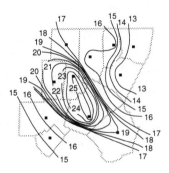

Population Potential (000)
Population Aged ≥ 75

Data Source: US Census of Population, 1990.
Produced by: NC Rural Health Research Program, Cecil G. Sheps Center for Health Services Research,
UNC - Chapel Hill.

minium complexes), the "points" for which population is counted and from which it is measured could have more distance within them than between them. For example, the distance between two buildings on a map may be less than one millimeter, which could have the analogous effect of making the distance within the "point" building less than that between buildings. Changing the scale of measurement or changing to real-world measures of distance instead of map analogs can solve the problem. Analysts must be cognizant of potential pitfalls and adjust appropriately for these factors.

This section has been concerned with measures of population distribution and examples of common dimensions of population have been mapped by locational quotients, demographic bases, and population potential. Comparison of their representations of distribution should suggest a variety of usages appropriate to each. One might, for example, construct demographic base maps to illustrate need or assess coverage for "Meals on Wheels" programs, transportation for handicapped individuals, or influenza vaccination of the elderly. Shading of a proportion of each unit could be used to illustrate the proportion living alone, disabled, or at special risk due to age. A population potential map could be constructed for a preschool population to assess the potential of disease diffusion, to determine the most accessible locations for day care facilities, or to identify optimal locations to access information or vaccination programs. Social activity cells—used to depict areas of routine, daily activity for specific subgroups of the population—could be used to identify the distribution of older teen exposures and areas of social risk and information circulation. The possibilities are essentially endless.

Population Mobility

Population mobility at the local scale affects age-, sex-, and race-specific exposure to environmental hazards and access to health services, while mobility at regional or national scales affects the (population) denominator of rates—greatly complicating the study of disease etiology when population exposures over long periods of time are involved. A variety of data sets (which are generally difficult to work with) exist for studying migration. For example, there is a special sampling of social security files to track migration. However, for most purposes planners and researchers turn to the US Census. The decennial Census captures geographical mobility as movement to a different house in the same county, to a different county of the same state, a different state, or a different region, as well as individuals returning from outside the United States. Population circulation, or micro-mobility that does not involve changing residence, is reported as commuting.

Macro-mobility trends

The mobility changes of the 1980's included an overall decline in migration to 18 percent of the population (from 20% in the 1950's and 1960's) despite an increase in the proportion of the population in the most mobile age group, 20 year olds (US Bureau of the Census, 1991). Non-farm households moved at a higher rate than farm households (22.1% compared with 15.11%), and white and black homeowners moved at similar rates (7.4% versus 7.6%). Although white renters were more mobile (35.6% compared to 29.2% for blacks), a higher proportion of blacks rented so that their overall mobility rate was higher (20.0% compared to 16.7%); a full quarter of Hispanics moved, but again that was due to a higher proportion renting rather than different owner or renter mobility rates. In general, the pattern of migration resembled previous decades more than the 1970's.

In the 1970's, the long-term trend of national concentration and local deconcentration ended. The nation deconcentrated as population moved to noncontiguous, nonmetropolitan areas. The three major types of nonmetropolitan destinations were energy and mineral development sites, recreational destinations, and new retirement destinations (Brown & Beale, 1981; Lichter et al., 1985; Morrill, 1988). In the 1980's, the nation as a whole returned to metropolitan growth; even in the South as a whole, nonmetropolitan counties returned to net outmigration (Forstall, 1991). The nonmetropolitan counties that grew most clearly were ex-urban or contiguous with existing metropolitan regions.

The 1980 Census recorded a great change in the migration pattern of the country. For more than half a century, the three great sweeps of population had been from the center of the country to the coasts, from the South to the North, and from rural to urban and then metropolitan areas. In that decade, the North lost population to the South, sparking many studies of "return migration." Even more dramatic was the historic turnaround that saw rural counties, non-contiguous to metropolitan, grow while most metropolitan areas lost population. The 1990 Census shows that rural and most nonmetropolitan population net growth has ceased.

From 1980 to 1990, the metropolitan population grew by 20 million or 1.1 percent annually, compared with nonmetropolitan growth of 2.1 million or 0.4 percent annually (Forstall, 1991). Although the metropolitan population reached a record 77.5 percent, the absolute number of nonmetropolitan residents grew. Notwithstanding this growth, 8 of 12 states in the Midwest experienced nonmetropolitan population loss. In the South, the least metropolitan region, population growth throughout nonmetropolitan areas has fallen from 1.5 percent annually in the 1970's to 0.5 percent in the 1980's with net outmigration by the end of the decade for the first time since the 1960's (Forstall, 1991). Although regional disparities have decreased, the metropolitan populations of the West and, at a decreasing rate, the South have continued to grow more rapidly than the Midwest or the recovering growth of the metropolitan Northeast.

As can be seen from Figure 3-6, the popular notion of mass migration at time of retirement is a myth. Mobility decreases with age after its peak in the early twenties. Fewer than 6 percent of people aged 65-69 moved between 1989 and 1990, and half of them moved within the same county. Only 0.15 percent of people aged 65-69 and 0.32 percent of those aged 75-79 moved from outside a metropolitan area to a metropolitan area; 0.41 percent and 0.22 percent, respectively, moved from a metropolitan area to a non-metropolitan area (US Bureau of the Census, 1991). Although the Northeast remained virtually stable, with 0.04 percent of 65-69 year olds moving both into and out of metropolitan areas, the South continued to see a net movement of this age group to nonmetropolitan counties from metropolitan ones (0.3% in to, and 0.54% out of metropolitan counties) and a net shift into metropolitan areas after age 75. Most nonmetropolitan retirement destination counties continued to grow. While the mobility rates for seniors are low, they still translate into tens of thousands every year seeking nonmetropolitan residences, mainly in targeted retirement areas.

There can be little doubt that retirees have an impact upon their destination areas, but their specific impact on health services remains unclear. Transfer payments from state and national levels through Medicare and Medicaid bring some limited support with older people independent of local taxes. Retirees are both attracted to recreation areas with service-based economies and themselves demand services, rather than goods, resulting in poorly diversified local economies characterized by low-paid employment opportunities and concomitant population growth. Thus, retirement destination counties are growing in several ways but the proportion of elderly persons may not significantly increase. Most in-migrating retirees are young-old and in fairly good health. The relative impacts on specific health service needs, specific disease prevalence, and the cost benefits of retirement upon destination areas are areas of active research by the National Institutes of Health.

One study which sought to address some of the questions concerning the impact of elderly migration was conducted in seven counties along the South Atlantic Coast (Bennett, 1990). Less than four percent of the retired households in any of the counties used the ambulance service and one percent utilized home health care during the year. Hospitalization was most often nonemergent and retirees could choose between local and other state and national facilities. Less than one-fifth of retired households thought they might need home health care or nursing home care within five years; however, between one-third and one-half thought they would eventually move out of the county—mostly because of illness or incapacitation of one of the spouses. Even though the retirees bought medicine through the mail and travelled out of the county for treatments, a quarter to a third in each of the counties spent at least $100 a month locally on medicine. In the older settlements, more than half spent $1,200 or more a year on doctors and hospitals, but younger retirement areas spent little. Some retirees complained of shortages in local medical personnel but this was mainly true for specialists such as cardiologists versus physicians in general.

Some of the impacts of population mobility on health conditions and demand for services can be summarized by returning to the population pyramids of Figures 3-7 and 3-8. The pyramid for Sweetwater County, Wyoming shows a population that was booming in the 1980 Census from young adult in-migration, mainly for oil and mineral development. In 1990, they are ten years older, their children are of school age, the small population cohort that got jobs after them—perhaps born in the county—are having children, and there are few elderly because the population used to be small. The pyramid for Marion County, Florida, shows the impact of retirement in-migration as well as the increase in service employment and business opportunities for young adults and their children. The impact of mobility on age structure, and consequently on morbidity and mortality and health service demands, can be projected and analyzed using the techniques discussed in this chapter.

Micro-Mobility

Micro-mobility involves the movement or circulation of people at the local level as well as at daily or weekly time intervals. It includes the journey to work, journey to school, shopping, recreational activities, local visiting, etc. The spatial pattern of such activities is important for accessibility to health services and to information dissemination (as well as in the spread of infectious disease). The social activity areas of teenagers, for example, involve not only the network of their social contacts but the space in which they occur and in which information or services may or may not be present. One way to analyze such activity areas is by means of the standard deviational ellipse (SDE), which encloses an elliptical area that includes approximately two-thirds of all of a target population's movements.

Standard Deviational Ellipse

Geographers are interested in making sense out of spatial patterns of all sorts. One technique of summarizing patterns of points is the standard deviational ellipse (Yuill, 1971). The SDE allows for the graphical representation of the average location, dispersion, and orientation of a set of points on a two-dimensional, x-y coordinate space. Raine (1978) outlines four steps necessary to calculate the SDE. These are:

1) calculating the mean center of gravity, also known as the bivariate mean;

2) calculating the standard deviation along the x axis from a coordinate system set over the mean center of gravity;

3) rotating the axes through a constant interval and calculating new standard deviations; and

4) joining the standard deviations to form the ellipse.

Several measures are then possible after the ellipse is constructed. The area and number (value) of points within the ellipse provide a measure of concentration one standard deviation around the mean center of gravity. The ellipse allows for the measurement of the shape, as a coefficient of circularity, and orientation in degrees, away from a specified axis. In usual practice the vertical axis is chosen, though in certain circumstances another axis might be more appropriate.

What makes this technique so useful is that several ellipses can be compared rather easily for differences or similarities in area, point count, orientation and shape. Still, there are important limitations to this technique. The first is the restriction of shapes to ellipses regardless of the actual shape of the distribution. The second is that the shape of the ellipse can be influenced by the shape of the study area. If the point distribution is away from boundaries and in only a portion of the study area, the impact on the shape of the ellipse is minimal. If the points are distributed throughout the study area, this will have a significant impact on the shape of the ellipse. A question then arises to which there is no consistent answer: how much of the shape of the ellipse is caused by the distribution of points and how much by the shape of the study area?

Risks Specific to Rural Areas

The other way in which local mobility is important is in the determination of who is exposed to what risk for how long. There are several risks unique, or at least more common, to rural areas: wells may be polluted by fertilizers; people outdoors may be affected by air sprayed with insecticides; farm, underground fuel, and chemical tanks may leach into aquifers; animal fecal contamination may affect swimming or drinking water. A second set of hazards is posed by vectored diseases, especially those such as Lyme disease or Rocky Mountain spotted fever, which have natural animal population foci (and tick vectors) that people or their pets contact more frequently in rural conditions. A third set of hazards is posed by rural roads, which together with rural vehicles and rural drivers, claim high levels of vehicular accidents and mortality. For all·these risks and more, it is the micro-mobility of the population that determines who (of what age or sex or race) is exposed at a certain place and time to a certain kind and level of disease risk. Standard deviational ellipses can again be used to determine the size and directional bias of the territory over which people are moving. Population potential maps (discussed earlier in this chapter) can be created for hazards. Having people recall their movements over the past twenty-four hours can be used to augment this to analyze time–space patterns of population exposure. This reported information can then be displayed using SDEs.

Two final kinds of population mobility are important for special exposures and risks: tourists and migrant workers. Tourism is a part of population circulation which exposes people from outside the area to local risks (e.g., ticks, rabid raccoons, plague-infected ground squirrels), introduces disease agents from outside the area (e.g., influenza, AIDS), and through sickness and accidents places demand on local health services (e.g., bus or airplane crashes). Unless tourism is at reliably high levels each year, it is difficult to include in any planning because it introduces a wild card.

Migrant labor constitutes a different degree of hazard since migrants are not only exposed to all of the above types of hazard but to local water and chemical risks as well. Fecal contamination of water in camps, exposure to tuberculosis, and introduction or spread of various parasites can all vary spatially with the paths and prevalence of migrant workers. Micro-level regionalization for exposures as well as service access can facilitate intervention and planning.

Small Area Projection and Planning

The age structure and other aspects of population composition can be analyzed spatially using techniques described above. Population can also be "survived" from year to year by applying local birth and death rates. Numerous microcomputer software products exist for constructing pyramids and for computer mapping if the scale is relevant. An example of a relatively easy-to-use computer package designed to produce population pyramids is IPSS® (Interactive Population Statistical System) from PSRC Software in Bowling Green, Ohio; see the Technical Notes for additional information. Manuals and programs for "small area analysis" became in high demand in the 1980's, and methods have been well documented and disseminated (US National Institute of Mental Health, 1989). Most states have agencies which disseminate the latest state estimates of local population numbers and composition. The states, and any interested researcher, can get current data and estimates of mobility, composition, marriage, childbirth, mortality, and more from the ongoing reports provided by the *Current Population Reports* of the US Bureau of the Census.

The composition, distribution, and mobility of population along the rural–urban continuum have profound impact upon disease patterns and service needs. Spatial analysis of population patterns can be simply and cheaply done for many purposes such as analyzing disease etiology, disseminating information, and regionalizing emergency and other local service needs. However, the caveats brought out in this discussion should be appropriately addressed to ensure accurate evaluation and analysis of population trends for use in meeting the health service delivery and disease treatment needs of a population.

▷P O I N T
▷OF DEPARTURE

Data Sources for Health Services Research
Lucy A. Savitz and Lise K. Fondren

Health services research relies heavily upon the use of secondary data. This is information that has been collected by someone other than the researcher(s) and frequently for another purpose. For example, a state bureau of labor may collect employment and unemployment statistics at the county level in response to a need to anticipate tax revenues or unemployment payments. These data could be used by health services researchers to predict the proportion of a county's population that is covered by commercial or private health insurance for all counties in a state.

There are two primary advantages cited for using secondary data to answer research questions. These are: 1) they provide timely results, and 2) they are relatively inexpensive (Kiecolt & Nathan, 1985). Both of these features relate to the fact that the data have already been collected and presumably verified and edited as well.

Since secondary data are usually collected for another purpose, they can potentially create several problems in health services research. For example, erroneous conclusions can be drawn because the analysis ignores complex sampling, the data are compared to a nonrepresentative population, or the data may have been collected for reasons so different from the present research question that there is no logical link. Each of these will be briefly discussed.

Sample Errors. To determine whether or not special procedures adjusting for incorrect standard errors are warranted, one should check the sampling design employed to collect the secondary data being used. Available documentation should be reviewed to ensure that the sampling design and the universe are known before using secondary data. Surveys like the Current Population Survey and the National Medical Expenditure Survey use complex sampling designs that over-represent certain subgroups of the population. If these datasets are used for other analyses without adjusting for these sampling variations, incorrect standard errors may occur, leading to confidence intervals and statistical significance tests that are incorrectly under- or over-stated. This creates the potential for erroneous conclusions. More thorough coverage of these procedures is discussed by Landis et al. (1982), DuMouchel and Duncan (1983), Lee et al. (1989), and Korn and Graubard (1991).

Computer programs such as SUDAAN™ can be used to correct the standard errors and calculate the design effect introduced by the sampling frame. If the researcher is only interested in the parameter estimates from a regression analysis or in a calculation of descriptive statistics and comparative ratios (e.g., relative risk) without consideration of statistical significance testing and/or confidence intervals, then provided weights can be applied when performing the procedure(s) of interest in most computer statistical packages.

Important questions any researcher should ask when using precollected survey data include: Was a random sample used? Who was (in)eligible for inclusion? Did the original researchers over-sample for certain characteristics (e.g., race, income, gender, Census region, rural or urban residence, voting district)? Recognition of potential problems and appropriate correction allow the use of precollected survey data to remain a viable, timely, and economical option for health services research.

Comparison with Nonrepresentative Populations. A frequent problem occurs when a researcher attempts to compare disease or utilization rates among or between populations. Often, state or national rates are used as a benchmark in ascertaining excess "risk" for a particular sentinel event. A direct comparison may be inappropriate because of varying racial mixes among the referent and comparison areas. For example, comparing a high infant mortality rate for a county which is predominately non-white with another county or region which is predominately white would be problematic given that nonwhites, overall, have higher infant mortality death rates. Crude (unadjusted) rates can be standardized or adjusted either directly or indirectly to eliminate the problem, allowing for a more appropriate comparison. The Point of Departure accompanying Chapter 8 discusses and illustrates these techniques. These issues are further discussed in the *Population Dimensions* (Chapter 3), *Contagious Diseases* (Chapter 8), and *Evaluating Clusters* (Chapter 9) chapters of this book.

Data Appropriateness. Health services researchers may also find themselves faced with the situation where they can identify an available secondary dataset that is pertinent to their research interest, but encounter problems because certain variables are unavailable or have not been measured in the optimal form. This can be discerned by carefully viewing the data collection instrument and/or documentation before using secondary data. When the variable of interest cannot be found, proxy variables, or variables that approximate the influential variable of interest, can possibly be used.

Data may also be collected categorically rather than continuously; for example, income might be reported within certain ranges—less than $5,000; $5,000-$15,000;

POINT OF DEPARTURE

P
O
I
N
T

O
F

$15,000-$25,000, and more than $25,000. These income data would have been more useful if they had been collected as a continuous variable, asking people for their family incomes rather than an income range, since the ranges used do not match Poverty Guideline thresholds nor are they amenable to various poverty classifications given the large category at the upper bound. The ranges are an impediment to a researcher wanting to tie income to various poverty levels based on the federal poverty guidelines. Researchers confronted with problems of this type are left to cope, identifying limitations in their reported results, or to search for other data sources.

How to Locate Usable Secondary Data

D
E
P
A
R
T

T
U
R
E

There are numerous sources of secondary data. The most common sources include government agencies, other research projects, insurers, trade groups or associations, and licensing or regulatory agencies. We will list some of the common sources available for health services researchers in each of these categories.

Government Agencies. State, federal and some local governmental agencies are a rich source of low cost and/or free secondary data. An afternoon of telephone calls or library research can usually uncover pertinent reports that present useful cross-sectional and time series data that can be compiled to create a database or used to answer basic research and policy questions. While the official names and organizational structures may vary from state to state, health, demography, and labor departments are easy to track down. Several important classes of data available from these sources include population data and projections, (un)employment data, income, environmental, basic infrastructure (e.g., roads, hazardous waste site locations), descriptive data concerning health care resources and availability, basic information on regulated insurers, social and human services data such as Medicaid and Medicare, and health data, e.g., disease incidence/prevalence, mortality and morbidity statistics, fertility and birth rates, and injury rates.

Some states also support registries to track health care problems like cancer (see Chapter 9) and immunization; no national database is currently available for these. Also, more than half of the states now support inpatient databases that collect clinical, cost, facility, and basic demographic information for acute care hospital discharges. Some of these also collect outpatient data as well. The National Association of Health Data Organizations is a valuable resource (NAHDO, 254-B North Washington Street, Falls Church, VA 22046) for contact information including a complete listing of those states with legislative mandates to gather hospital-level data. Also, Fry and Young (1992) provide a state-by-state inventory of health care data with contact information. Many commercial organizations prepare data from governmental agencies for distribution. Other direct federal sources for leads on secondary data availability are listed at the end of this Point of Departure. This is by no means intended to be a comprehensive listing. A more thorough listing, *Health Information Resources in the Federal Government*, Fifth Edition, 1990, has been prepared by the Office of Disease Prevention and Health Promotion National Health Information Center (PO Box 1133, Washington, DC 20013-1133). The National Library of Medicine has produced a useful book entitled *Health Services: Sources of Information for Research* [NLM-PSD-92-01] (1992) that contains a section on statistical sources and includes sources of both tabular and computer-readable data. We also recommend Appendix I to *Health, United States, 1992* (US NCHS, 1993), put out by the National Center for Health Statistics, for an excellent discussion of sources and limitations of data.

Other Research Projects. Contacting other researchers interested in similar issues and/or identifying them

POINT OF DEPARTURE

through published literature searches can be a reasonable source of secondary data. In these instances, collaborative arrangements may be made to conduct additional analyses of an existing dataset. The National Center for Health Statistics also produces a *Catalog of Electronic Data Products From the National Center of Health Statistics* (1992), which describes available datasets. Many major health insurers conduct research studies; they may be willing to collaborate with researchers investigating issues pertinent to their operations. Also, the Pew Charitable Trusts has provided funding to the Foundation for Health Services Research together with the Cecil G. Sheps Center for Health Services Research to create and maintain a database of ongoing publicly and privately sponsored research projects in health services research for the US. This database is known as *HSRProj*. Further information can be obtained from Marian Mankin at the Foundation for Health Services Research at (202) 223-2477.

Trade Groups, Associations, Licensing Boards and Regulatory Agencies. Many trade groups and organizations collect information about their members. For example, state medical societies, nursing organizations, and hospital associations may be used to access important data critical to a research investigation. Fry and Young (1992) list contacts for each state's hospital association. The Point of Departure *Tracking Doctors into the Twenty-First Century* in Chapter 5 discusses the importance of data from physician trade associations. Groups such as these may be the only source of information for other health professionals such as physical therapists and chiropractors, while state licensing boards and regulatory agencies may be of assistance when searching for data on nurses, physicians, dentists, pharmacists, and certified nurse midwives.

In this discussion we have tried to briefly discuss the advantages of, some common problems with, and leads in locating secondary data for health services research. The importance of secondary data in addressing policy issues, generating hypotheses for future research, investigating health problems, and targeting intervention/education programs should not be underestimated. However, it is the responsibility of researchers to ferret out potential limitations of secondary data in terms of their quality, appropriateness, and means of measurement when using them as a basis for continued study.

Federal Data Source Contacts:

Bureau of Economic Analysis
US Department of Commerce
1441 L Street, NW
Washington, DC 20230; (202) 606-9900
A good source for basic economic and labor data for the nation.

Bureau of Health Professions, Information Officer
Health Resources and Services Administration
Parklawn Building, Room 8-05
5600 Fishers Lane
Rockville, MD 20857; (301) 443-5794
Distributes fact sheets, trend reports, and study results. Data requests will be forwarded to the Office of Health Analysis and Research.

Centers for Disease Control, Public Inquiries
1600 Clifton Road, NE
Atlanta, GA 30333; (404) 639-3534 for publications
Maintains disease surveillance information through data collection, analysis, and laboratory investigation.

Environmental Protection Agency
Public Information Center
MC-3404, 401 M Street, SW
Washington, DC 20460; (202) 260-2080
General publications available for a wide range
of topics.

National Center for Health Statistics, Data Dis-
semination/Publications
Centers for Disease Control
6525 Belcrest Road, Room 1064
Hyattsville, MD 20782; (301) 436-8500
A primary data source for information needed to
monitor the year 2000 objectives as well as a
resource reference for other data and methodological
information.

Health Care Financing Administration, Public
Affairs Office
200 Independence Avenue, SW, Room 423-H
Washington, DC 20201; (202) 690-6113
This agency administers the Medicare and Medicaid
programs; cost report data and provider information
are available from this primary source.
For statistical data: Baltimore office (410) 597-
3934.

National Cancer Institute
Office of Cancer Communications
Public Inquiries Section, Building 31, Room
10A24
9000 Rockville Pike
Bethesda, MD 20892; (301) 496-5583
Publications on cancer-related topics are available.

National Maternal and Child Health Clearinghouse
Information Specialist,
8201 Greensboro Drive, Suite 600
McLean, VA 22102; (703) 821-8955, ext. 254 or
265; fax: (703) 821-2098
Centralized source of information on maternal and
child health.

National Institute of Environmental Health Sciences, Office of Communications
P.O. Box 12233, WC-03
Research Triangle Park, NC 27709; (919) 541-3345
Information and research findings concerning
environmental exposures.

US Bureau of the Census
Customer Services, Room 326-WPI
Washington, DC 20233; (301) 763-4100;
fax: (301) 763-4794
OR Contact your local regional office for information about population, demographics, insurance,
work travel, location information, and many other
variables collected in the decennial census.

POINT OF DEPARTURE

Chapter 4

Access to Health Services

Point of Departure:
Access and Cartography

In this chapter we focus on the geographic aspects of access and give examples of methods for measuring access, or its absence, using geographic and spatial approaches. Before describing the geographic characteristics of access, we discuss in some depth the concept of access, a concept that has figured prominently in policy decisions concerning the allocation of health care resources and the implementation of programs to change the way physicians are trained, hospitals are organized, and ambulatory care services are delivered. The question of what constitutes "adequacy" in access has been important for many years, especially for rural communities which are typically considered to have lower levels of access to health care services. We suggest that measures of access can be approximated in several ways based on spatial aggregations and metrics grounded in a spatial ordering of resources.

I. Access as Concept

Access to health services has received quite a bit of attention in the literature over the past 30 years. This was due to a desire by policy makers to understand those factors that could be altered administratively or through policy action to improve accessibility and to produce some desired outcome (e.g., better health status, reduction in infant mortality). Initially, investigative attempts to measure accessibility to health services were plagued by the absence of two common features: 1) a basic model that described the complex relationship of variables pertinent to the study of health care access; and 2) a generally accepted definition of access which could be operationalized.

At the symbolic level, access may seem to be a simple, uniformly agreed upon social goal. There are many policy statements that focus on access as the most appropriate goal for the American health care system (President's Commission, 1983). Operationally, however, access is a very complex construct where many nuances and levels surface when attempts are made to analyze specifically what access is. Conceptually, access is simple in that it reflects many of our concerns about the fairness of the health care system, combining our national beliefs in equal opportunity and our sense of social responsibility to those less fortunate. We believe that Americans are endowed with specific, equal rights spelled out in our laws and the Constitution, as well as a smaller number of implied rights based on the courts' interpretations of those laws (the right to privacy is an example). When considering the distribution of commodities and services, we feel that rather than a right to simply receive material resources, we have an equal opportunity to earn them. Following this logic, equal *opportunity* with regard to health is often translated into equal *access* to health services.

Access is closely allied with the concept of quality of care. Common markers of disparities in access and/or the quality of accessible care are sometimes called sentinel health events, events which include preventable diseases, disabilities or untimely deaths, and whose occurrence serves as a signal that the quality of or access to preventive and/or therapeutic medical care may need to be improved (e.g., maternal death; Rutstein et al., 1976). The complexity of access arises when we introduce the term as a formal part of our health policies.

A. Modeling the Concept of Access

In 1968, Ronald Andersen and colleagues (1975) published a behavioral model of families' use of health services, which hypothesized that there were three basic sets of factors related to an individual's decision to seek and use health care services: predisposing factors that existed prior to the onset of illness, enabling factors that related to the ability to secure services, and need for medical care. This model focused on individual behavior and the identification of influential variables which could be targeted for interventions designed to increase an individual's ability to utilize health care.

While Andersen's behavioral model made a valuable contribution to our understanding of accessibility at the family level, the model required expansion to facilitate the study of access or medical care from a delivery system perspective. This expanded version, which is commonly referred to as the Framework for the Study of Access (Aday & Andersen, 1974), moves the theoretical focus from the individual to populations. The Framework states that "access may be defined as those dimensions which describe the potential and actual entry of a given population group to the health care delivery system." Aday and Anderson sought to develop and test a model that could empirically describe access. Their elaborated model added notions of *potential* and *realized* access and included national and professional policies in the framework. Thus, aspects of federal and state health financing would be included as predisposing variables that could partially describe the potential access of a population in combination with individual or aggregate measures such as age, sex, race, and attitude toward illness. The enabling characteristics of personal income, mobility, and insurance coverage would then be added to provide a composite picture of the potential access for a population. The realized access measures described actual use of services and satisfaction with those services, and, when combined with measures of need, a specific metric of appropriate access could be constructed. Two measures were constructed: the Use Disability and Symptoms Response ratios, which used expert opinion to build a scale that indicated whether a person with a given set of restricted activities or symptoms made appropriate use of health services.

The Aday and Andersen framework was used in two large-scale evaluations of primary care initiatives. The first, a national evaluation of rural primary care programs, surveyed organizations and local users and non-users of the target clinics to measure potential and realized access (Patrick et al., 1988). That analysis found that the two were neither well-correlated nor consistent in several important instances. Adults scored high on potential access indicators, and low on realized access; the opposite was true for the children. The second evaluation, of the potential for hospitals to deliver community-based primary care, was limited by the number of cases and no conclusive confirmation of the model was offered (Shortell et al., 1984).

More formal criticism of the Aday and Andersen model was voiced by Roy Penchansky (1977), who pointed out that a single concept of access really couldn't hold together and advocated more specific areas that could be measured as factors that showed more consistent correlation in empirical studies. Those factors include: availability, accessibility, accommodation, affordability, and acceptability. Penchansky and Thomas attempted to verify this model for access (1981) but based their conclusions on an analysis of a relatively small sample of homogenous employed persons in one region of the United States. The Penchansky-Thomas approach did not receive the attention of the Aday and Anderson model but holds some attraction from a geographic perspective in that it proposes that the use of specific measures be closely tied to spatial distributions. The use of the Gini index and other variants was proposed to measure inequality in the availability of resources. In the accessibility dimension, indices were based on distance and travel time, perceived distance, and opportunity costs. The utility of either the Aday and Andersen or the Penchansky approach has not yet been conclusively demonstrated, but the latter's use of geographic concepts makes it more congruent with the methods described in this volume.

Nonetheless, both the Aday and Andersen comparisons of realized and potential access and Penchansky's five dimensions can be displayed in a geographic context, using cartographic methods such as difference maps or overlays of data with boundary maps; examples of these methods as applied to indicators of access related to vaccine coverage are included in this chapter's Point of Departure, *Access and Cartography.*

B. Access as "Coverage"

A notable difficulty with the Aday and Andersen conceptual model is that it tends to atomize the study of access by dividing any analysis into component parts according to their framework. These parts are conceptually linked within a unified, causal network. However, because empirical work has not supported this pattern, the model does not fully explain the concept of access. Similarly, by segmenting related aspects of accessibility, Penchansky's dimensions also lead to fragmentation. An alternative to these approaches is to look at access in a more unified way.

One way to do this is to look at access as a continuum of "coverage," meaning the proportions of people who can use, do use, and effectively use health services. In this continuum, proposed by Hongvivatana (1984), access can be seen to have many levels— from availability of services to actual "appropriate" delivery and use of those services. Figure 4-1 illustrates access envisioned as a continuum of coverage. The different levels of coverage allow us to direct policy and research questions to the specific factors that affect access at one or more levels. The underlying assumption is that the policy maker will wish to frame program goals in terms of access at a particular level on the vertical axis. Even if policy makers in the United States were to declare equal access to health

Figure 4-1
Access as Continuum

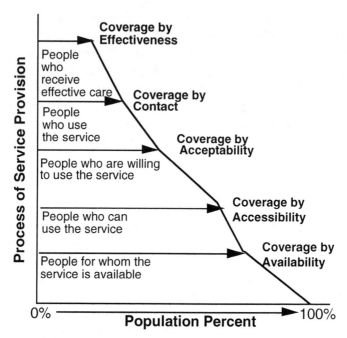

Source: Hongvivatana, T. 1984. Data analysis: Social science perspective. In: *Evaluating primary health care in southeast Asia, proceedings of a regional seminar.* New Delhi: Regional Office, World Health Organization.

care services to be a right, we would have to decide at what point along the vertical continuum we were willing to ensure access.

II. Geographic Aspects of Access

Analysis of access at the operational level is complex, embracing many interrelated factors and/or barriers. A geographic or spatial analysis of access tends to focus specifically on access in terms of availability (or relative location of consumers and points of medical care delivery as well as distance traveled). In discussing the general concept of access, Aday and Andersen (1974) differentiate between geographic and socio-organizational access, wherein geographic accessibility "refers to the 'friction of space' that is a function of the time and physical distance that must be traversed to get care and socio-organizational attributes include all those attributes of the resources, other than spatial attributes, that either facilitate or hinder the efforts of the client to obtain care." Studies of spatial availability patterns in rural areas tend to more comprehensively capture access since geographic distance factors far outweigh other factors such as income, education, illness level, and values and beliefs (Joseph & Bantock, 1982; Thouez, Bodson & Joseph, 1988). This may reflect a basic problem with a concept like access: its meaning and usefulness vary based on factors such as geography.

We will discuss measures of access as they have been used in geography. The basic uses have been measures that focus on: distance, ideal ratios for defined populations, small area variations, vector analysis, inequalities, spatial effectiveness, and spatial interaction. These divisions of the empirical methods used to examine access are somewhat arbitrary; each overlaps the other to some degree and one approach may be combined with others. However, each approach has unique aspects; we will discuss some of those below.

A. *Distance*

Distance to care is an important, yet often overlooked, issue in health services research. It is known to be a barrier to access (Donabedian, 1973; Joseph & Phillips, 1984). Distance to care has been used both to independently measure access and availability and as one of many factors in the study of health care utilization (Joseph & Phillips, 1984). Hospital service areas are often constructed using data based on the residence of patients who have sought care at a particular facility or using a radius to define a population whose residences fall within a specified boundary (Morrill & Earickson, 1966; Garnick et al., 1987; Morrisey et al., 1988; Wright, 1990). Distance has been shown to be an important factor in utilization (Shannon et al., 1969, 1979; Morrill & Earickson, 1968; Morrill, Earickson & Rees, 1973; Mayer, 1983; Williams et al., 1983; McGuirk & Porell, 1984), but measures of distance have often been crude or replaced by proxy variables because of cumbersome data requirements and/or cartographic limitations.

Joseph and Phillips (1984) reviewed the various measures of distance—travel time, linear distance, and road mileage—and expanded the notion of geographic accessibility to include location (physical proximity) and effective accessibility (whether a facility is always available or open and whether a person's time–space budget permits her/him to use the service) by borrowing from an earlier discussion of geographic accessibility by Donabedian (1973). Another measure of distance that is particularly relevant when considering health care accessibility is that of perceived distance. For example, rural residents, who are accustomed to traveling long distances, may view a trip length of 50 miles very differently than urban residents would. Consumers of health care services are likely to act upon perceived rather than real distances (Winter, 1986). The Minkowski Metric (Sneath & Sokal, 1973) measures the distance between two points (e.g., a hospital and a patient's residence), but includes a factor that can be adjusted for perceptual differences. Unfortunately, the adjustment requires external data inputs. See the inset at right, *Calculating the Minkowski Metric*, for more detailed information.

Friction of Distance. Economic geography posits that consumers tend to use those services located nearest to them. This is based upon: 1) the concept of spatial interaction, referring to the movement of goods and services and people across space, and 2) the principle of least effort, based on the assumption that one minimizes distance and selects the shortest path when moving between two points, which accounts in a general way for the length and intensity of this movement. Underlying the principle of least effort is the idea of friction of distance, which incorporates the resistance to movement over space. This has been used to demonstrate variable distance decay for medical services, whereby patients are willing to travel different distances for varying levels of service (Mayer, 1983; Gesler & Cromartie, 1985). This observed inverse relation-

Calculating the Minkowski Metric

The Minkowski Metric may be calculated as follows:

$$d_{i,j} = \sqrt[r]{(x_i - x_j)^r + (y_i - y_j)^r}$$

where $d_{i,j}$ is Minkowski's distance between points i and j;

x_i, x_j are the x coordinates of points i and j;

y_i, y_j are the y coordinates of points i and j; and

r is the exponent and 1 / r th root used to measure distance.

The r factor can be used to adjust for exaggerated perceptions in distance; for example r = 1 can indicate a city block and r = 2 linear distance (as the crow flies). The larger the exponent, the greater the weight placed on perceptual differences in distance. For individuals perceiving distances to be double their actual length, an r value greater than 1 is needed to model this phenomena; however researchers have argued that the r value should be set at something other than 2 (Appelbaum, 1966; Huff, 1963, 1966). Regression results suggest that r = 1 is suitable for health care facility locations that one actually utilizes and r = 3 is most appropriate for distances to competitive facilities (Winter, 1986). Selection of the appropriate r value(s) is left to the analyst or researcher to determine, given the particular question at hand and the limitations of available computers, software, and databases.

ship between distance and type of service is described as a linear decrease in the probability that an individual will use a medical service. The relationship is dependent upon the type of service, and varies within service categories by subgroups of the population, as well as by other factors that determine utilization, e.g., race, age, income, education, and other patterns of service consumption (shopping behavior, or regularly traveled pathways to work and recreation, i.e., activity spaces (Meade et al., 1988)). In general, consumers are willing to travel longer distances for specialized services (e.g., organ transplantation, cancer treatment, trauma care) than for more routine services (e.g., general physical exams, ear infections, minor injuries).

Standards and thresholds for distance traveled. Spatial or geographic considerations in access to care relate to any person who must travel some distance to reach services. In the development of the Graduate Medical Education National Advisory Committee (GMENAC) Report, a special panel devoted to geographic considerations attempted to develop standards for access to services based upon distance to care expressed as travel time. Table 4-1 summarizes their general recommendations (Graduate Medical Education National Advisory Committee, 1980).

The recommendations of the Geographic Access Panel were not acted upon in any specific way, and there has been very little work done to verify or support the times-to-service standards recommended by the GMENAC panel. The National Rural Health Association (NRHA) together with the Frontier Health Care Task Force described distinguishing characteristics of service areas defined by population density (Elison, 1986). Urban residents (more than 100 persons per square mile) generally have a less than 30-minute driving time to reach a large, group practice with specialty care and where a high level of technology is accessible; rural residents (more than six but fewer than 100 persons per square mile) most often have a 30-minute drive to reach a small, group practice staffed by a generalist who has occasional specialist consultations on site and easy-to-moderate access to a medium level of technology; and frontier area residents (fewer than six persons per

Table 4-1
GMENAC Standards for Geographic Access

	GMENAC Modeling Panel Adjusted Needs Based Range of Ratios of Physicians by Specialty per 100,000 for 1990	Minimum Acceptable Ratio for All Areas [1/]	Range of Times to Service/ Manpower	Recommended Times to Service/ Manpower
Emergency Medical Services	5.3-5.7	2.7-2.9	5-30 min.	30 min.
Obstetrical Services (OB/GYN)	18.4-20.0*	9.2-10.0*	30 min.-1 hour	45 min.
Child Care/ Pediatric Medical Care	47.1-51.2**	23.6-25.6**	30 min.-1 hour	30 min.
Adult Medical Care (FP/GP/ Internal Medicine)	26.7-30.8 (IM); 33.2-35.7 (FP/GP)	13.4-15.4 (IM); 16.6-17.9 (FP/GP)	20 min.-1 hour	30 min.
Surgical Care/ General Surgery	9.4-9.8	4.7-4.9	30 min.-2 hours	90 min.

1/ One-half of GMENAC Modeling Panel needs-based estimate.
* Per 100,000 women of all ages
** Per 100,000 children under 17
Adapted from Table 5, p. 63; Report of the Graduate Medical Education National Advisory Committee to the Secretary, Department of Health and Human Services, Volume III, Geographic Distribution Technical Panel, 1980.

square mile) normally have a 60-minute drive and may experience severe geographic and climatic conditions during their drive to reach a generalist, primary care group and/or mid-level practitioners, all of whom tend to have infrequent specialist consultations and difficult access to even a low level of technology.

B. Population Requirements for Various Service Levels

Several advocates of regionalized systems, including Fry (1971), Mountin et al. (1942), and the Committee on the Costs of Medical Care (1972), proposed an ideal geographic distribution of health care services (facilities, personnel, and administration) based on the size of the population serviced. In geography, these approaches are termed *population potential* and *regionalization*. Higher order services (e.g., specialty care such as neurology) are only available in more populous places; generalist care is more commonly available in less populous places.

In reality, resource distribution is far from ideal. Joseph and Bantock (1982) concluded from their study of physician distribution that simply increasing the supply of physicians can actually increase the maldistribution of physicians in favor of urban places. The trend toward specialization and larger group practices, which increases the population threshold necessary to economically support a practice, has been found to further increase this divergence between rural and urban areas (Northcutt, 1980). To counter these trends, advocates for rural constituencies have proposed minimum standards of service accessibility for rural and frontier populations. The Frontier Health Care Task Force and the National Rural Health Association developed minimum recommended health services for service areas of varying population size (Elison, 1986; see Table 4-2). The model they propose does not incorporate the relative dispersion of population or specify the sizes of the service areas. These could have been accounted for by tying the service areas to a measure of population density—the ratio between population size and land area (typically square miles). Population densities range from very dense (urban areas) to very sparse (frontier areas). A related concern is population dispersion or the size of the land area over which a population is spread. The lack of sufficient population to support the existence of certain service levels and the need for financial subsidization are critical issues in large, sparsely populated areas; nevertheless, the need for health care services varies

Table 4-2
Minimum Recommended Health Services

Population / Service Area	EMS	Primary Care	Specialty Care	Hospitalization
less than 500	First Responder EMT B-P	Intermittent MLP or MD by appointment; Satellite/part-time clinic; EMT supervision via telecommunication and written protocol	Referral	Referral
500-900	EMT B-P First Responder network in outlying areas	Full-time MLP or part-time MD; arrangement for emergency coverage and EMT supervision	Referral or periodic arrangement in the community	Referral
900-1,500	EMT B-P First Responder network	Full-time MD or MLP, or combination full- and part-time group practice; emergency coverage and EMT supervision	Referral or periodic arrangement in the community	Referral and infirmary model
1,500-4,000+	EMT B-P First Responder network	Small group practice; combination of MD and/or MLP; medical specialists (MD/MLP); IM, PED or OB, CNM as determined by community need; emergency coverage and EMT supervision	On-site full-time regularly scheduled clinic within primary care practice, or referral	Small community hospital or infirmary referral

Source: Elison, Gar. 1986. Frontier areas: problems for delivery of health care services. *Rural Health Care* 8:5, p. 3.

little by a person's geographic location in that a pregnant woman in an urban area has medical care needs remarkably similar to those of a pregnant woman living in a very remote, frontier area in Wyoming.

The definition of frontier. The notion of frontier is uniquely American and is interwoven into the cultural perspective of the nation (Popper, 1986). It is also a term that describes the large variation in population density in the United States. Its formal use in policies reflects the need to consider certain areas of the nation separately with regard to health care delivery programs (Hewitt, 1989). Frontier areas, according to convention, are those counties with population densities of fewer than six persons per square mile. These are the most remote areas in the United States and are located almost exclusively in the western United States and Alaska. Geographic distances between towns are great, implying small-scale analyses over large land areas. For frontier areas, the population standards often do not meet minimum criteria for allocation of resources. Even the most necessary services such as emergency and obstetric care must be justified using alternative approaches to a regional hierarchy.

C. *Small and Other Area Variations*

In determining whether a population or a geographic area has or does not have access, resources are compared to needs. Ratios of providers to population are commonly used to indicate relative access. Aday and Andersen included outcome measures as part of their framework, but in the time between their publishing and the present, little use has been made of their realized access measures. There has been recent work that re-focuses attention on outcome measures based upon observed variations in use of services and the connection between certain types of use and related implications for access.

The phenomenon of small area variations in rates of surgery and hospitalization has prompted much study into the reasons for the variation and has led to the search for general standards of care (Wennberg, 1984). The fundamental assumption in the analysis of small area variations is that wide differences reveal a pattern of potentially inappropriate care. There is, however, no complete consensus on whether differences in rates reflect too much or too little care (Leape et al., 1990). The differences between communities in rates of utilization, hospitalization, and surgical and diagnostic procedures are sometimes striking. These differences reflect real differences in the way medicine is practiced, but we cannot determine if those differences are due to inappropriate use of services. The "enthusiasm hypothesis" wherein geographic differences in utilization are caused by differences in the prevalence of physicians who are 'enthusiasts' for particular services has been proposed as an explanation (Chassin, 1993). Wennberg also suggests that there may be different theories of medicine or different levels of uncertainty in the practice of medicine that cause these differences.

Uncertainty over the degree to which one or another rate is appropriate for specific procedures suggests that it will be exceedingly difficult to determine what rates are appropriate for primary care. Many studies of the appropriateness of particular clinical strategies produce conflicting results; nevertheless, it is clear that the best understanding of variations comes from the study of large samples of patients and clinical decisions (Diehr et al., 1990). This suggests that large-scale studies of primary care content and primary care outcomes are required in order to determine what the optimal range of appropriate practice will be to ensure effective access. It is interesting to note that the most complete published review (Paul-Shaheen et al., 1987) of the small area analysis literature uses an earlier version of the Aday and Andersen access conceptualization (Andersen & Newman, 1973) to organize the discussion of practice variations, a topic that has become very important in health care policy.

Given the intense attention paid to the relationship between use of services and outcomes, it was almost inevitable that outcomes themselves would be used as indicators of use, or, in a policy sense, as indicators of access. John Billings (1990) has suggested that small area variations might indicate differences in levels of access for population groups. Billings found that admission rates for selected conditions varied in relation to income for the ZIP code areas he examined using 1984 and 1987 hospital discharge data for New York City. He found that cases that were "Ambulatory Care Sensitive" showed a variation related to income; this implied that lower income patients were subject to access barriers for this type of care. This ambulatory care sensitive measure was also used by the Codman Research Group (1991) for its study of access to rural hospitals. Generally Billings and the Codman Group found significant differences in most discretionary treatment according to the income of the small areas, but no differences for emergency utilization.

D. Use of Vectors

Vectors are used to depict directional flows—flows of goods and services across an area. For health services research purposes, they serve as a visual summarization of health care seeking behavior, population mobility, and physician referral patterns, among other uses. While simplistic, they are a powerful and flexible way to graphically display information and indicate patterns of actual use and access as use.

Vectors are derived from some measure of frequency of use between two points (e.g., patient county of residence and Hospital A). One of the first uses of this tool in the literature was to evaluate rural consumers' health care seeking behavior in southern Utah (Kane, 1975). Francis and Schneider (1984) present several good examples of the variety of uses a particular facility might make of this technique in examining five years of data for cancer patient flows in Washington. The development and advances in computer-assisted cartography or mapping have made vector analysis much more available.

Figure 4-2 presents a vector map depicting patient flows to acute care hospitals in Mecklenburg County, North Carolina. While this example focuses on patient flows from county of residence to facility of inpatient admission, vectors can also be used to depict a variety of categorical values (e.g., willingness to travel). Temporal and cross-sectional comparisons are possible. Note that the width of the vector or arrow can be used to reflect the relative size of the flow since the thickness of the arrows allows a visual comparison of a variable.

E. Measures of Inequality

The Gini index is a tool used primarily by social scientists to measure the level of inequality in the distribution of a resource

Figure 4-2
Vector Map Showing Inpatient Migration

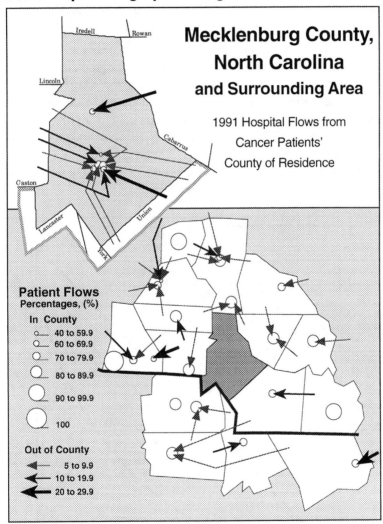

Data Source: South Carolina Department of Health and Environmental Control; North Carolina Medical Database Commission. Data compiled from reported 1991 figures.

within a given population, its classic application being the measurement of income distribution. Figure 4-3 describes the generalized application of the Gini index and the Lorenz curve, the geometric interpretation of most calculations of inequality.

While physician-to-population ratios have utility as indicators of physician availability within a specific geographic area, the overall ratio tends to mask variation, and the examination of individual ratios becomes difficult when trying to compare the distribution of ratios across many subunits if there are more than a few. Morrow (1977) and Gogan et al. (1979) were among the first health services researchers to study the level of inequality in the geographic distribution of physicians nationwide and in individual

Figure 4-3
Generalized Gini Index

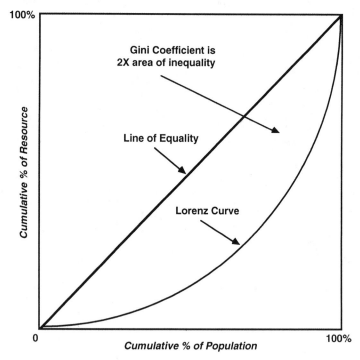

states by using the Gini index. Morrow's comparisons of the distribution of medical personnel in the United States from 1906 to 1974 by specialty, occupation, and market area using Gini indices suggested a maldistribution of primary care physicians nationwide. Using North Carolina data, Gogan et al. compared the supply and geographic distribution of physicians in selected counties with similar counties across the United States and showed that North Carolina counties had a greater "unevenness" in the geographic distribution of physicians than all other US counties from 1970 to 1976. They concluded that there was no indication of improvement in the geographic distribution of physicians in the counties studied from 1970 to 1976, despite the fact that the supply of physicians was increasing statewide. More recently McConnel and Tobias (1986) compared changes in Gini indices for the distribution of physicians among specialties by aggregating them into metropolitan areas and all counties.

An analysis of the geographic distribution of primary care physicians for selected years between 1975 and 1988 by the Sheps Center for Health Services Research suggests that, as measured by the Gini index: 1) general/family practice physicians exhibited the greatest equality in geographic distribution, but they were the only primary care specialists whose distribution worsened across almost all county categories; 2) among all primary care physician specialists, obstetricians/gynecologists exhibited the greatest inequality in geographic distribution; 3) there has been an improvement in the distribution of pediatricians, obstetricians/gynecologists, and general internal medicine physicians but substantial variations still exist among different categories of counties; 4) generally, metropolitan counties had a more equal geographic distribution of physicians than nonmetropolitan counties; and 5) within the subcategories of metropolitan and nonmetropolitan counties, the more populous counties tended to have a more equal distribution of physicians than the less populous counties (Study of models, 1992). These results indicate that the overall availability of family and general practitioners in the population has fallen while the supply has risen. (See Chapter 5, *Health Professions Distributions*, for more detailed information on calculating the Gini index.)

F. Spatial Effectiveness

Joseph and Bantock (1982) developed an index to calculate the potential spatial access of communities to the medical care delivery system in the area. This index is useful in that it can be disaggregated to compare patterns among various subgroups of the population being examined, depicting differences in the utilization of medical care. However, this index approaches access from a limited standpoint, focusing on spatial separation while ignoring the other relevant dimensions of access that have been previously discussed. This measure was further developed by Thouez et al. (1988) to overcome these basic limitations through a regression-based application that estimates the overall potential spatial effectiveness of the health care delivery system in overcoming distance barriers. Application of this extended measure is presented in the *Health Professions Distributions* chapter (Chapter 5). The major advantages of these measures are their relative ease in application and minimal data requirements.

G. Spatial Interaction Model

Cowper and Kushman (1987) developed an interesting spatial interaction model that they used to analyze the primary health care seeking behavior of rural consumers. This type of model evaluates the flow of goods and services (in this case, health care services). The model was estimated using a large, three-county area in northern California. This was a large-scale, data-intensive effort, requiring data on individuals, consumer origins, facility utilization, and care site locations that may not be readily available for generalized applications of this method. Nevertheless, the value of the model lies in its usefulness in simulating and predicting the impact of changes in the health care delivery system of a given region (e.g., hospital closing, physician retiring).

This section has highlighted several basic geographic techniques that can be used to measure access to health care. It is not intended to be comprehensive but rather to stimulate interest in the use of these tools. One other notable methodological techniques deserves mention: the standard deviational ellipse, which measures individual activity spaces and can be useful in understanding health care consumers' choice of providers for medical care. The use of standard deviational ellipses is covered in greater detail in Chapter 3.

III. Emerging Questions in Access

Improving access to health care has been part of almost every call for reform of the health care system in the recent past. Policy makers and politicians set goals for access which may not be able to be evaluated when new programs are implemented. Health care delivery is becoming more regionalized or, more precisely, is concentrating into a number of urban places with clusters of high-technology services. This trend is spurring calls for a structured division of the nation into areas where health plans or health financing cooperatives will be allowed to compete or to gain monopolies (depending on their structure and the particular policy that is adopted). The obvious disciplines that may help policy makers guide this phenomenon are geography and health services research. Some may see this as a revival of the planning activities that briefly flourished in the 1970's and, in large part, it is. But there is a fundamental difference in the pressure for action in the 1990's: the need for geographic analyses now comes from the need to improve the efficiency of markets in order to restrain the overall costs of care rather than as a pretense for forcing geographical analyses on immature market systems. Geography has a long tradition of examining market activity and has applied that to health services. Determining what constitutes access and where access may be less than optimal are tasks that geographic methods can achieve.

Access as a concept is enjoying yet another resurgence in interest in the first half of the 1990's. The Committee on Monitoring Access to Personal Health Services of the Institute of Medicine began work in 1990 and released its report, *Access to Health Care in America*, in 1993. That study calls for outcomes-based indicators of access, i.e., measures of access that are reflected in the disease structure of a community. Much of the approach advocated in this report comes from the "Social Indicator Movement" that gained popularity in the 1960's and was refined in the health care field through the development of "sentinel events" (Rutstein et al.,

1976), clinical conditions that would normally be preventable and that occur when there is a lack of timely primary care. John Billings, in his work with the United Hospital Fund of New York, further developed this type of approach to monitoring the performance of a health care delivery system. Billings related small area socioeconomic data to the occurrence of "ambulatory sensitive conditions" and found that higher occurrence of these conditions was correlated with income and race. This type of health data monitoring related to populations is being proposed as one way to measure the quality of care in a reformed health care system. Assessment of outcomes is tied to access in the conceptual model proposed by the Institute of Medicine, but there has been little discussion of the geographic aspects of the access–outcome relationship (Millman, 1993).

Geographic criteria in access and performance standards attempt to incorporate the relationship between distance and care-seeking and care-giving behavior. The tools presented in this volume provide some means by which these relationships can be explored. The challenge to the health services research community is then to take up these methods to address the policy problems which will emerge with the allocation of areas for regional health plans or alliances and the need to identify areas of underservice and need.

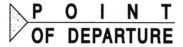

P O I N T
OF DEPARTURE

Access and Cartography
Lucy A. Savitz and Don Albert

Hypothetical Example, Real Circumstances

A health department in a county is concerned about immunization status of two-year-old children. They want to use funds from a major health initiative to most effectively target areas for educational intervention efforts for this important preventive care service. The National Vaccine Advisory Committee listed inadequate access as a primary barrier to appropriate immunization in terms of: 1) lack of a primary health care provider, 2) financial constraints to well-child care, and 3) failure of private insurance to include immunizations as a covered service (Freed et al., 1993). Immunization of preschool-aged children has become a major area of interest given very low estimates of immunization coverage, the large number of working mothers placing their children in day care, and recent outbreaks of preventable disease. The *Healthy People 2000* report (US DHHS, 1990) specifies a national goal of 90 percent of all children having completed the basic series of immunizations by their second birthday. This goal has been revised to reflect changes made in the basic immunization series and incorporated into the state's health care objectives, which are monitored at both the local and state levels.

In an attempt to monitor and target programmatic intervention efforts, a difference map is first constructed at the Census tract-level using population data from the US Bureau of the Census or the state demographic database in combination with data from the state's (hypothetical, for purposes of this example) central immunization registry.[1] The first map shown here (Figure 4-4) displays patterns in the difference between the actual number of two-year-old county residents at Time A and the number of two-year-old residents who have been appropriately immunized by their second birthday in Time A, based upon current immunization guidelines (4 doses of diphtheria and tetanus toxoids with pertussis vaccine or DTP; 1 dose of measles, mumps, and rubella or MMR vaccine; 3 doses of oral polio virus or OPV vaccine; 3 doses of Hepatitis B; and 4 doses of Hibs). More simplistically, Figure 4-4 displays the number of two-year-old children not properly immunized, with the darker shading showing higher numbers of children without complete immunization. Figure 4-5 indicates the percentage of children without complete immunization. Such a display presents an objective indicator of realized access.

This difference map displays a snapshot of immunization coverage among a subset of the child population where higher values reflect larger gaps and no difference indicates complete, appropriate immunization coverage. Conclusions should be drawn with caution because results may be overstated and comparisons of differences over time may be inappropriate due to changes in immunization guidelines. For a long time, the "basic series" remained stable; however, recent vaccine developments have caused recommendations for the basic series to be changed. Simple differences also have an inherent weakness in that they don't reflect relative magnitude—Census tracts with a difference in population of two for an age group comprised of 4 persons (50%) and a population of 400 (0.5%) are

[1] Reliable immunization data are not readily available at any level at the time of this writing; however, some state and local efforts to construct immunization registries and national sample data collection efforts are currently underway given the Clinton Administration's interest in this public health issue.

Figure 4-4 **Children Two Years Old Without Complete Immunization: Number**

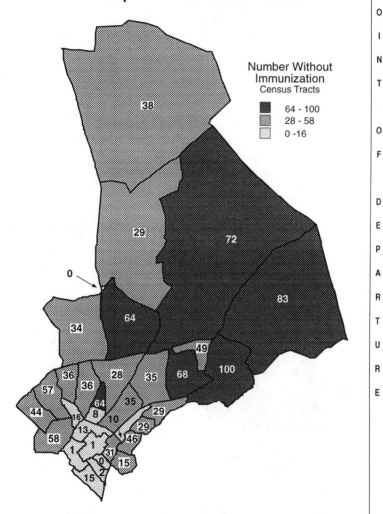

Number Without Immunization
Census Tracts

■ 64 - 100
▨ 28 - 58
□ 0 -16

P
O
I
N
T

O
F

D
E
P
A
R
T
U
R
E

Data Source: This hypothetical map represents a continuum of urban, suburban, and rural Census tracts. The number of children aged two without complete immunization is shown within each Census tract.

Figure 4-5   **Children Two Years Old Without Complete Immunization: Percent**

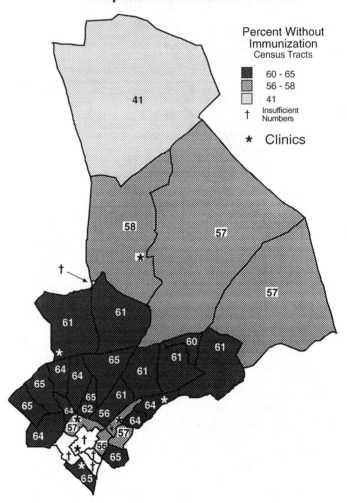

Percent Without Immunization
Census Tracts

- 60 - 65
- 56 - 58
- 41
- † Insufficient Numbers

★ Clinics

Data Source: This hypothetical map represents a continuum of urban, suburban, and rural Census tracts. The percentage of children aged two without complete immunization is shown within the Census tract.
Note: † denotes insufficient numbers to calculate a reliable percentage; most of these Census tracts are commercial or industrial.

similarly represented. Nevertheless, absolute numbers provide a useful beginning; however, percentages can be used to further distinguish areas of relative "need" (Figure 4-5). This difference map can be enhanced by producing an overlay map, which combines these differences (objective indicators of realized access) with overlays of information that are related to poten-

Table 4-3

Estimated Immunization Rates By Population Characteristics

Total	37-56%
Race	
White	41-60%
Black	20-33%
Area of Residence	
Urban	31-43%
Suburban	40-61%
Rural	42-62%

Source: CDC, 1994.

tial access for immunization coverage (e.g., process indicators such as population density, poverty status, and racial mix; or a structural indicator such as primary care provider location). Racial mix and rural/urban estimated immunization ranges were used to construct this example with data from the National Health Interview Survey (CDC, 1994). Estimates of immunization by race and area of residence can be used to give more detail to the map. Using the difference map, we have identified Census tracts with low levels of immunization coverage indicated by relatively larger difference values. The overlay map depicted in Figure 4-6 provides additional, related information about the at-risk population by simultaneously incorporating a relevant population characteristic (race) and the number of children without complete immunization as well as a geographic feature (clinic locations).

This map can then be used, for example, to target Census tracts where interventions through door-to-door canvassing might be valuable given the established,

POINT OF DEPARTURE

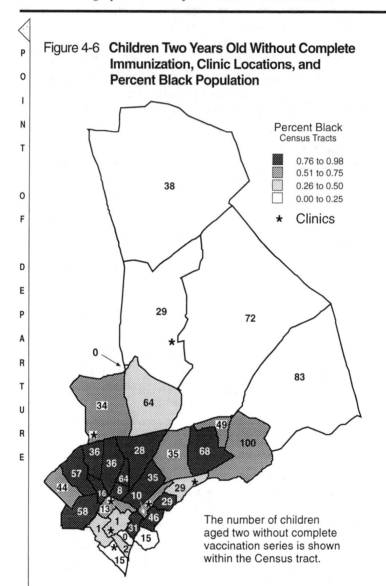

Figure 4-6   **Children Two Years Old Without Complete Immunization, Clinic Locations, and Percent Black Population**

Percent Black
Census Tracts

0.76 to 0.98
0.51 to 0.75
0.26 to 0.50
0.00 to 0.25

★ Clinics

The number of children aged two without complete vaccination series is shown within the Census tract.

Data Source: Hypothetical.

positive effect of educational efforts on increases in immunization coverage. Areas with large nonwhite populations may benfit from the use of nonwhite educators and/or special attention to cultural and logistic barriers (e.g., no providers) inherent in these areas. Figure 4-6 isolates problem areas within this hypothetical county by simultaneously presenting select indicators of both potential and realized access which distinguish differences in immunization coverage in order to identify areas appropriate for intervention.

The synthetic estimates used for the purpose of this example were generated using proportions from a national sample that were then applied to 1990 Census data. This hypothetical case was designed to demonstrate the utility of geographic analysis that may be possible with data that are beginning to be collected across the US. Awareness of possible uses of these data may also serve to guide the development of databases currently being compiled.

POINT OF DEPARTURE

Chapter 5

Health Professions Distributions

Points of Departure:
Community-Based Measures of Underservice
Tracking Doctors Into the Twenty-First Century

Introduction

This chapter examines the geographical distribution of people who are employed in various health professions. The location of practitioners with respect to patients and potential patients lends itself easily to cartographic displays of descriptive information and more complex spatial analysis. We are all familiar with maps and graphs that depict differences in the distribution of practitioners; choroplethic maps that show that there are more or fewer doctors or nurses in some counties or states than others are the most common. This type of display or analysis focuses on the *availability* of practitioners, which has become a major issue in health services research and health policy as we debate whether availability means access. Another issue which is closely related but explores the issue of distribution in a normative way is the question of whether the distribution of practitioners is *equitable*. The question of equity requires different analytic techniques than availability and depends upon some basic assumptions about preferences. These preferences must be clear to the analyst before data describing supply of health professionals can be interpreted.

In this chapter we illustrate approaches to the examination of professional availability by asking two specific questions: first, Are enough professionals of a certain type available in a certain area to adequately serve the area's population? This question brings up further questions about underservice, satisfying needs and demands, and geographic scale of analysis. The second question asks, Does the spatial distribution of health professionals provide for adequate physical accessibility? Here the main issues are various measures of distance between patients and providers and distance thresholds for various specialties.

In terms of equity, we are concerned with whether or not the same numbers of practitioners are available in different areas of a health care delivery region. Geographic scale of analysis and the role of specialties are again of importance here.

To introduce the more common approaches to using geography to display or analyze availability we will first present a single case study which will help to focus the reader's attention on a concrete situation. Later in the chapter we will discuss in more depth the problems and analytic complexities that arise in the study of health professional distributions. Then we will ask a series of questions arising from the case study and attempt to answer them. Finally, we will suggest and illustrate more advanced ways of measuring availability and equity.

Case Study: The Distribution of Oncologists in North Carolina

We decided to use oncologists in North Carolina as a basis for our case study for several reasons. Oncologists deal with one of the diseases of greatest concern to society, cancer. Cancer was the second leading cause of death in the United States for 1988, accounting for almost one-quarter of the deaths nationwide in that year. The American Cancer Society estimated that 1,130,000 new cases (excluding carcinoma in situ [100,000] and nonmelanoma skin cancer [600,000]) and 520,000 deaths would be diagnosed or attributed to cancer of all sites in 1992. The federal government has targeted breast and lung cancer prevention efforts in its *Year 2000 National Health Objectives.* In its "Cancer Control Objectives for the Nation: 1985-2000," the National Cancer Institute (NCI) set forth the goal of reducing cancer mortality by 50 percent by the year 2000—but pointed out the importance of addressing the needs of minorities given survival differences among ethnic groups in this country. There are some striking differences between African-Americans and whites in the mortality rates for certain cancers. For example, the mortality rate for cervical cancer during 1978-81 was 3.2 per 100,000 for whites, while it was 8.8 per 100,000 for African-Americans. In geographic terms, Greenberg (1983) and Monroe et al. (1992) have shown that, on the national level, rural mortality rates for many different cancers have been converging toward what were once higher urban rates. There is now little difference in cancer incidence between these two subgroups.

When we look at small areas like counties there are rate differences that show some rural places with very high rates and others with low rates. Given the differences due to scale, we should examine the availability of professionals at a level appropriate to the distributions of both the disease and the professionals who treat it. By describing, geographically, the distributions of rural populations by race, for example, together with the distribution of oncologists in the State of North Carolina we can illustrate many of the typical problems of scale associated with mapping health resource availability and equity.

Like many other specialists, oncologists tend to be clustered in densely populated areas. Some less densely populated areas of North Carolina may, therefore, have very poor access to these specialists. Regional comparisons of oncologist availability display some gross inequities. There are also different levels of oncological specialization, each with its own market area or population threshold. Furthermore, not all phases of cancer diagnosis

Figure 5-1   Oncologists By County, North Carolina, 1990

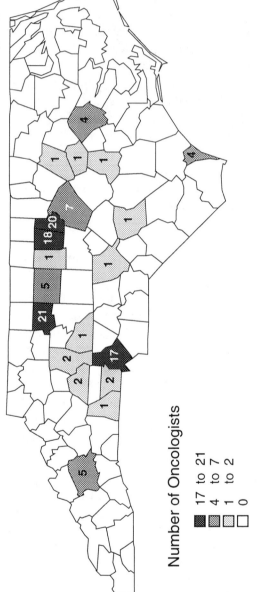

Number of Oncologists

17 to 21
4 to 7
1 to 2
0

The number of oncologists is
shown within county boundaries.

Data Source: 1990 NC Board of Medical Examiners Licensing Data, maintained by the Cecil G. Sheps Center for Health Services Research.
Produced by: NC Rural Health Research Program, Cecil G. Sheps Center for Health Services Research, UNC - Chapel Hill.

and treatment are performed by oncologists, and people are willing to travel different distances for different levels of treatment.

Figure 5-1 is a choroplethic map showing the number of oncologists in each of the 100 counties of North Carolina in 1990. This map basically identifies counties with oncologists, and gives some idea of the number in each county. As mentioned above, oncologists are concentrated in the more populous counties—out of 100 counties, 20 had at least one oncologist and 80 had none. A larger scale (e.g., ZIP code level) map would probably indicate even greater concentration in the physical distribution of oncologists across the state. We have not shown hospital location here, but it is closely related to the distribution of the specialists. The availability of cancer specialists depends upon their physical location; counties that are nearer to oncologists have those services more available than those counties that are farther away. Figure 5-2 adds information about counties with hospitals or comprehensive cancer centers which have one or more oncologist(s), and counties adjacent to counties with facilities having three or more oncologists.

Counties with a comprehensive cancer center or a hospital with three or more oncologists are called Level 3 counties. This particular means of classification was considered for use in an analysis of the proportion of cancer cases diagnosed at certain stages of development and the degree of availability of cancer specialists. It was felt that populations closer to specialists might have their cancers diagnosed earlier. The only location identifier for the cancer patients was the county and this classification scheme allowed for more subtle gradations of distance which, in this case, stood as a proxy for availability. There were only nine Level 3 counties. If a county was adjacent to a Level 3 county and was also in the service area of a Level 3 county (that is, if 10% or more of the county's resident, general hospital admissions were admitted to the adjacent Level 3 county hospitals), it was designated as a Level 2 county. About one-third of the counties fit into the Level 2 category. Counties with 1 or 2 oncologists at a hospital were called Level 1 counties. Only nine counties fell into this category. Level 0

Figure 5-2   **County Classification By Availability of Cancer Care, 1990**

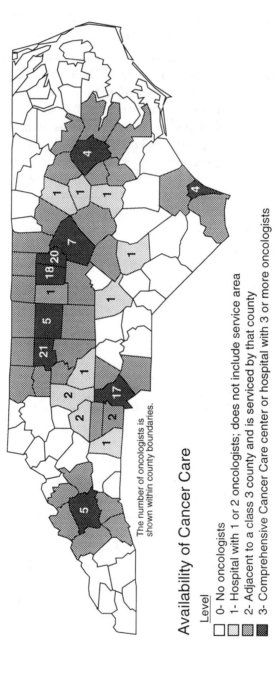

The number of oncologists is
shown within county boundaries.

Availability of Cancer Care

Level

0- No oncologists
1- Hospital with 1 or 2 oncologists; does not include service area
2- Adjacent to a class 3 county and is serviced by that county
3- Comprehensive Cancer Care center or hospital with 3 or more oncologists

Data Source: 1990 NC Board of Medical Examiners Licensing Data, maintained by the Cecil G. Sheps Center for Health Services Research.
Produced by: NC Rural Health Research Program, Cecil G. Sheps Center for Health Services Research, UNC - Chapel Hill.

counties had no oncologists or were not adjacent to counties that did; slightly over half the counties were in this category.

The spatial pattern of oncologists across the United States as in North Carolina is very uneven with several prominent clusters. That is not surprising, however, if one reviews the extensive literature examining the reasons why physicians, hospitals, and other health care resources are distributed in the way they are. The principle of central place theory (described in the *Glossary*) fairly accurately describes this phenomenon. Joseph and Phillips (1984) discuss three general categories of factors that cause concentrations in health services: economic (i.e., increasingly expensive treatments tend to create centralization of services); professional organization (i.e., increasing specialization and group practices); and government intervention (i.e., attempts to locate health personnel in rural areas). A substantial portion of this type of research has focused on the locational decisions of physicians and has found that, among other things, a community's population size, age structure, and racial composition, and the physician's medical school influences, lifestyle preferences, specialty, need for contact with colleagues, and orientation to health care facilities may be important factors in locational decisions. In North Carolina, for example, population and cancer care resources are concentrated in the Piedmont area in the middle of the state, only a small number of counties in the state contain a "large" city and/or a major hospital, and oncology is a specialty which requires a relatively large market area because cancer is a relatively rare disease (although cancer mortality rates are proportionally high).

It is clear from our maps that availability varies widely across the State of North Carolina, and that there are substantial intra-state inequalities. Some counties appear to be well served, while others have poor potential access to oncologists. Health planners and policy makers at different levels—state, regional, and local—may be quite concerned about this situation.

Questions Arising from the Case Study

Availability

Despite the usefulness of the maps in Figures 5-1 and 5-2, they fail to tell us about many important details, and we may pose further questions. Oncologists are concentrated in the Piedmont part of the state, but so is the population; therefore, to some extent, need and demand might be in balance with supply. This notion suggests that we need to look at oncologist-to-population ratios. Figure 5-3 displays ratios of oncologists to total population by county. There is some problem in interpreting this map because 80 percent of the counties had no oncologists in 1990, but we can still make some interesting comparisons among the counties that did have oncologists. What stands out is that, although the map does relate supply to need, there are still inequalities when population is taken into account. Most of the counties with large hospitals—Buncombe, Forsyth, Orange, Durham, Pitt, and New Hanover—have the lowest oncologist-to-population ratios (greatest supply in relation to population). Thus, although Figure 5-3 provides more information than Figure 5-2, it can be improved upon further.

Cancer does not come upon members of subpopulations equally (for example, different age groups) and counties will vary in their age structure (see Chapter 3). Therefore, we should think about the *denominator* of the ratio more carefully—which segments of the population are most at risk from cancer? We should also recognize that different segments of the population will tend to require different subspecialties within oncology—a *numerator* concern. These considerations lead us to Figure 5-4, a map of ratios of urologic oncologists and surgical urologists to male populations over the age of 35. Here we intend to look at a specific cancer site—prostate cancer—and we have adjusted our parameters to give a more realistic match-up between supply and potential need or demand. The American Cancer Society predicted 34,000 deaths in the United States in 1992 from prostate cancer. Without clinical insight, it may have seemed obvious to include only oncologists in evaluating the availability of cancer care, but in North Carolina,

Figure 5-3 **Population Per Oncologist, 1990**

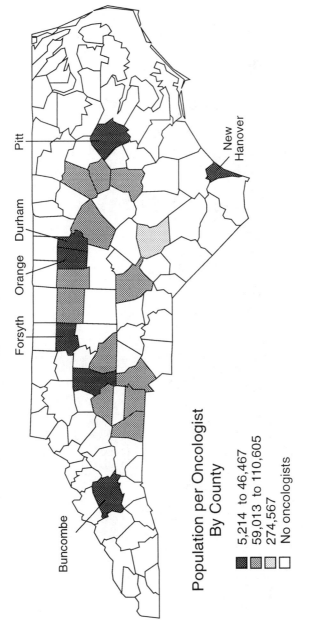

Population per Oncologist
By County

- 5,214 to 46,467
- 59,013 to 110,605
- 274,567
- No oncologists

Data Source: 1990 NC Board of Medical Examiners Licensing Data, maintained by the Cecil G. Sheps Center for Health Services Research;
1990 US Census. Produced by: NC Rural Health Research Program, Cecil G. Sheps Center for Health Services Research, UNC - Chapel Hill.

Figure 5-4   **Urologist-to-Population Ratios, 1990**

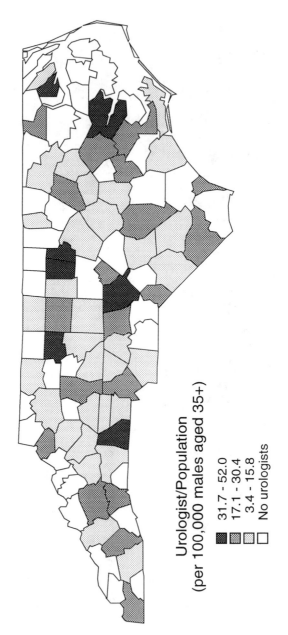

Urologist/Population
(per 100,000 males aged 35+)

▪ 31.7 - 52.0
▦ 17.1 - 30.4
▨ 3.4 - 15.8
☐ No urologists

Data Source: 1990 NC Board of Medical Examiners Licensing Data, maintained by the Cecil G. Sheps Center for Health Services Research; 1990 US Census. Produced by: NC Rural Health Research Program, Cecil G. Sheps Center for Health Services Research, UNC - Chapel Hill.

surgical urologists provide a significant proportion of care for patients afflicted with this particular cancer. Prostate cancer is a relatively common cancer that usually afflicts men over the age of 50. However, a review of North Carolina's incidence data from the state's Cancer Registry suggested the need to include men at younger ages because it also occurs in the under-50 male population. Figure 5-4 shows, as expected, high ratios of urologists in those counties with oncologists (some of whom are urologic oncologists), but the inclusion of surgical urologists spreads the availability of prostate cancer treatment over a much wider portion of the state. The spatial pattern in Figure 5-4 also reflects the distribution of the male population over 35 throughout North Carolina. There are still underserved regions in all sections of the state; clusters of several counties with no urologists exist in both the western mountains and along the eastern coast.

Equity

In Figures 5-5 and 5-6 we turn from a focus on availability across North Carolina to the issue of equity among different regions of the state. We selected Area Health Education Center (AHEC) regions as they represent a health service-oriented regionalization (see Chapter 6) specifically constructed to address issues such as the availability of physicians and other health care professionals.

Figure 5-5 shows a "raw data" pattern, using ratios of all types of oncologists to total population. The geographic pattern reflects the number of Level 1, Level 2 and Level 3 counties and their hospitals which lie within each AHEC region. There is a tenfold difference in ratios from the least well served to the best served AHECs. The Fayetteville, Eastern and Area L AHECs are clearly disadvantaged. Figure 5-6, like Figure 5-4, refines both the numerator and denominator to show intra-state inequalities. This map shows ratios of urologic oncologists and surgical urologists to male populations over age 35. In contrast to Figure 5-4, there is a more even spread of ratios across AHECs, with only a twofold difference between the highest and lowest ratios. This mainly reflects the addition of surgical urologists to the numerator.

Figure 5-5   **Oncologist-to-Population Ratios,   AHEC Regions, 1990**

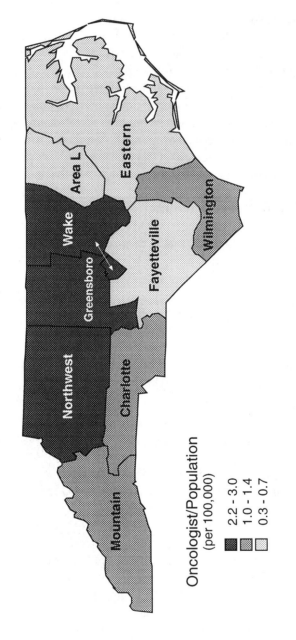

Oncologist/Population
(per 100,000)

■ 2.2 - 3.0
▦ 1.0 - 1.4
□ 0.3 - 0.7

Data Source: 1990 NC Board of Medical Examiners Licensing Data, maintained by the Cecil G. Sheps Center for Health Services Research; 1990 US Census. Produced by: NC Rural Health Research Program, Cecil G. Sheps Center for Health Services Research, UNC - Chapel Hill.

The initial map of the distribution of oncologists in North Carolina by county (Figure 5-1) raised questions concerning the relationship of people in need of oncology services to the professionals who can provide these services. The successive maps focused more and more on a particular relationship between the two, adding information as we went along. This progression answered a chain of questions but at least two more remain. How does the distribution in one area compare to that in other areas and the state as a whole? How equitable or inequitable is the distribution?

Availability Issues

The availability of medical personnel and facilities to consumers is one of the major issues in the US health care system today. The issue is particularly acute in specific geographic areas, such as remote rural places and poor inner-city areas. Despite a series of government-sponsored programs over the last several decades (Gesler, 1992) and the claims by researchers that increases in physician supply in the 1970's increased availability to many smaller communities (Williams et al., 1983; Newhouse et al., 1982a), the problem of inducing providers to locate in many chronically underserved areas remains.

Types of Availability

The most basic availability question is: what do we mean by the term itself? We refer here to two aspects of availability: a) the number or amount of resources with the potential to provide health care, and b) their distribution in space. Two other ways of describing the spatial component are to talk about the location of populations relative to health care resources and potential physical access.

Relation to Accessibility

Discussions of accessibility have indicated that availability was at the bottom of the access continuum (see Figure 4-1 in Chapter 4). Specific health care resources may be available to 100 percent of a population—that is, the resources are there—but they are usually not

Figure 5-6 **Urologist-to-Population Ratios, AHEC Regions, 1990**

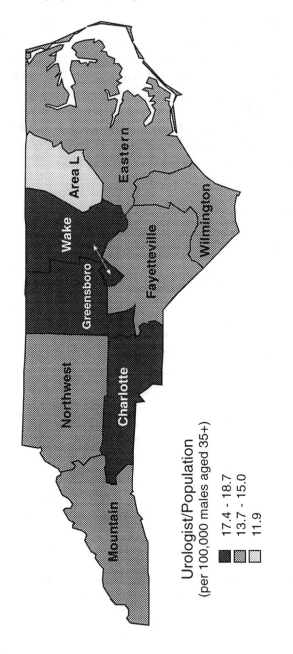

Urologist/Population
(per 100,000 males aged 35+)

■ 17.4 - 18.7
▨ 13.7 - 15.0
▨ 11.9

Data Source: 1990 NC Board of Medical Examiners Licensing Data, maintained by the Cecil G. Sheps Center for Health Services Research; 1990 US Census. Produced by: NC Rural Health Research Program, Cecil G. Sheps Center for Health Services Research, UNC - Chapel Hill.

accessible to everyone, are acceptable to even fewer people, and are actually used by or effective for fewer people still. We are obviously interested in utilization and effectiveness, but a fundamental task is to ensure that the services are available in the first place.

Numbers

Underservice

The various oncologist-to-population ratios we developed for Figures 5-1 through 5-6 are easily calculated, using data which are readily obtained from specialty societies or state licensing boards. But how do we know when particular populations are being well served or underserved? As Wysong (1975) points out, this is a deceptively easy question to ask. "Medical underservice" or "health services scarcity" may mean different things to different people (planners, health personnel, consumers) in different places. Attempts to define and operationalize these terms run into many difficulties. The Index of Medical Underservice, for example, does not define "underservice," nor does it distinguish between underservice and other concepts such as availability and accessibility. It is in reality a numerical expression based on four weighted variables that measure different aspects of the health care system: the ratio of primary care physicians to populations as an indicator of supply, the infant mortality ratio as an indicator of health status, and percent below poverty line and percent 65 and older as indicators of socioeconomic status. The quest for measures of underservice has resulted in the development of several measures for targeting communities for health professions placement programs and other subsidies to improve the supply of practitioners. The Index of Medical Underservice is only one of those. A brief review of others is included in the Point of Departure at the end of this chapter on *Community-Based Measures of Underservice.*

Needs and Demands

Questions of setting thresholds for availability often center around population needs and demands. Demand and need, of course, can be very different. And both are difficult to measure.

Need can be measured in many ways. Joseph and Phillips (1984), for example, differentiate between 1) *normative need*, which is determined for individuals by professionals, 2) *felt need*, which is expressed by individuals themselves, 3) *expressed need*, which leads to a demand for service, and 4) *comparative need*, which is professionally determined for certain population subgroups.

However we look at need, we generally require some information about population characteristics as different population subgroups require different types and levels of service. We recognized this fact in our cancer specialist examples when we modified the denominators in our oncologist-to-population ratios in Figures 5-4 and 5-6 to include only populations at greatest risk, based on a single population characteristic, age. But other variables are also important including race, sex, and income, as well as a variety of cultural traits such as illness beliefs that can identify individuals or groups who may be predisposed to certain negative health outcomes. Furthermore, there are factors other than population characteristics to consider. What about risk factors stemming from physical and man-made environments? Levels of potential environmental carcinogens are obviously germane to our case study. (These are considered in greater depth in Chapter 9.) There are also local attitudes toward health care to consider.

One way to determine if availability corresponds to need or demand is to compare practitioner distributions to the factors we have just been discussing by placing them on the same map. Figure 5-7 shows what happens when a map of urologic oncologists and surgical urologists is overlaid with a map of prostate cancer incidence for the Mountain AHEC. The map can be seen as a refinement of Figure 5-4, but here we have adjusted for variations in the age distribution of the population. This was accomplished indirectly using observed-to-expected ratios.

In comparing cancer incidence rates among the Mountain AHEC counties, it was necessary to adjust for age because the age distribution of the populations in these counties tended to be skewed. We chose the state population distribution as a "base" (national or regional distributions could be used depending on the disease being considered). Example calculations are shown for Henderson County in Table 5-1.

Observed state cases are divided by the state population for each age category under consideration to arrive at age-specific incidence rates. These are then multiplied by the county population in each age group, yielding expected cases. The number of expected cases is summed and observed county cases are divided by calculated expected cases in computing the O/E ratio. The critical cutoff is 1.0, where observed cases equal expected cases. Above 1.0, risk increases and county cases are higher than expected. Below 1.0, the risk of the cancer in the county is less than the state average. It is useful to think about the magnitude of effect as well. For example, there were 60.99 expected cases of prostate cancer and 83 observed cases for an excess of about 22 cases in Henderson County with a 1.36 O/E ratio. Swain County had a similar O/E ratio of 1.39 with an excess of fewer than three cases (7.17 expected cases and 10 observed cases). While the O/E ratio represents higher risk in Swain County, the magnitude of effect is quite different. Evaluation of the data at this level may be useful for public health agencies targeting intervention programs.

We've mapped the O/E ratio for each county within the Mountain AHEC region in Figure 5-7, with values in the range 0.8 to < 1.09 serving as the baseline (which is theoretically equal to 1.0) where observed incident cases equal calculated expected cases. Values above 1.0 suggest a higher incidence of prostate cancer than would be "expected" and values lower than 1.0 suggest a lower incidence of the cancer. Those counties with the greatest disparity between observed and expected cases do not have any providers and the two counties with lower than expected O/E ratios both have providers. Buncombe County, with the greatest number of care providers for prostate cancer, has an elevated ratio with 18 incident cases more than would have been expected (Observed–Expected). While incidence data add important information to the analysis, caution should be used in evaluating the spatial patterns because of

Table 5-1
Calculation of Adjusted Observed-to-Expected Ratios for Henderson County, North Carolina

Age Groups	State Prostate Cancer Cases	State Population	State Prostate Cancer Incidence Rate	Henderson Co. Population	# of Expected Cases in County	# of Observed Cases in County
35-39	2	258,741	0.000008	2,391	0.02	
40-44	4	235,204	0.000017	2,350	0.04	
45-49	13	186,750	0.000070	1,949	0.14	
50-54	50	152,039	0.000329	1,624	0.53	
55-59	144	138,660	0.001039	1,614	1.68	
60-64	358	133,553	0.002681	1,912	5.13	
65-69	638	120,981	0.005274	2,262	11.93	
70-74	715	86,147	0.008300	1,812	15.04	
75-79	618	57,509	0.010746	1,224	13.15	
80-84	345	30,680	0.011245	734	8.25	
85 +	217	18,391	0.011799	431	5.09	
Total	3,104	1,418,655		18,303	60.99	83

O/E 1.36

Figure 5-7 **Prostate Cancer, 1990**
Males 35+, Mountain AHEC

Observed/Expected Ratio
Indirectly Adjusted

☐ < 0.8
▦ 0.8 - 1.09
▨ 1.1 - 1.29
■ ≥ 1.3

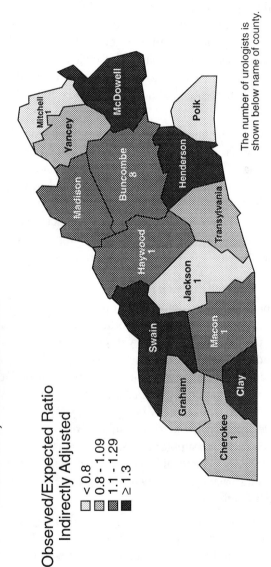

The number of urologists is
shown below name of county.

Data Sources: 1990 US Census, STF1A; NC Cancer Registry, State Center for Health and Environmental Statistics, Prostate Cancer, 1990; BME Data, October 1990, in "A Special Report on Health Care Resources in North Carolina" prepared by the Cecil G. Sheps Center for Health Services Research of the University of North Carolina at Chapel Hill. Produced by: NC Rural Health Research Program, Cecil G. Sheps Center for Health Services Research, UNC - Chapel Hill.

the variation within the shaded categories. For instance, Clay County and Henderson County are similarly shaded in terms of the O/E ratio but the magnitude of the effect is quite different because of the size of the population in these counties. There were three more incident cases observed than expected in Clay County and 22 in Henderson County. The magnitude of the effect should be taken into account in targeting public health funds and other policy initiatives.

While this map adds greater detail to our analysis, it still overlooks information that may be important. For example, it has been noted that there is higher mortality from and incidence of prostate cancer among blacks. However, it is unclear whether this may be a socioeconomic artifact where a comparison between poor blacks and poor whites would yield no major discrepancy in these rates. This analysis takes us into a level of complexity that makes cartographic display less than optimally effective.

Problems of Scale of Analysis

Many of the need and demand factors for health care have been identified. The problem is, their importance relative to availability varies from place to place. One very important conclusion reached in recent studies of rural and underserved populations, for example, is their diversity. This means that decisions about underservice require detailed community profiles rather than indices (Wysong, 1975). This approach is already being used by the US Division of Shortage Designation for its determination of HPSAs—they use locally provided data to supplement national data files in characterizing communities. The local input usually centers on the number of full-time-equivalent (FTE) physician and nonphysician primary care providers in the service area.

Mention of the importance of local variability gives rise to a further question: how local is local? In other words, what geographic scale should we be dealing with when we try to measure availability? The size of regions we choose "should be sensitive to changes in supply that affect access and utilization while at the same time avoiding a focus on single practitioners or practices" (Study of models, 1992). In addition, areas should be large enough to bring together sufficient resources to address specific problems. It has been shown that multi-county areas are the most rational scale for designating health care areas (see Chapter 6). Compare the county-level maps shown in Figures 5-3 and 5-4 with the AHEC-based maps in Figures 5-5 and 5-6. They tell different stories about availability. Different groups of people will have an interest in one set of maps or another. It would also be useful to have a national map with physician-to-population ratios by state so that North Carolina's oncologist availability could be compared with that of other states. Would a map showing ratios at a county subdivision level (e.g., ZIP code or minor civil division) be useful? Probably not for oncologist availability, given the market area or distance most people would be willing to travel to oncologists. So scale considerations relate in part to type of specialty. There were 115 oncologists in North Carolina in 1990 or an average of just over one per county, so perhaps the county or county cluster scale is appropriate for discussing their availability, although county-based maps may focus on single practitioners or practices and be distorted by the presence of a major teaching facility. On the other hand, there are 4,948 primary care physicians, or 495 per county, so their market areas are considerably smaller on average and, if we could obtain the appropriate data, maps based on county subdivisions might prove useful. The use of county averages in a situation like this one may be misleading because many of the geographic units (80 out of 100 in the case study) have no practitioners at all and outlier concentrations exist around medical schools which do not necessarily owe their location to population demand.

Need and Supply

The most typical method of examining the need for oncologists or other medical resources is to analyze disease prevalence and relate that to the existing number of providers, comparing the ratio to a standard. This is a procedure that captures situations at only one point in time, however. To study the effects of changes in availability over time requires further data. Patient survival data together with reliable incidence and prevalence data are optimal, but this information is usually not collected and is often unavailable on a timely basis if it is collected.

Alternatively, in the case of cancer, we could focus our attention on the stage of diagnosis. These data are collected by several states which have cancer registries that tabulate this along with incidence data, or by states participating in the Surveillance, Epidemiology and End Results (SEER) study sponsored by the NCI to estimate national rates of cancer and cancer treatment. Given the appropriate data, we could determine if incidence rates and mortality rates changed for various cancers as the availability of oncologists changed. For cancer and other chronic diseases, we would expect incidence to initially increase as a result of improved diagnosis capability and mortality to decrease due to increased survival afforded by care provided at earlier stages of diagnosis. One particular type of cancer may be particularly amenable to this type of longitudinal surveillance. Prostate cancer is becoming an important public health concern because there are improved methods of early detection while at the same time mortality rates are increasing. This type of analysis, however, can be confusing because other variables may be in operation at the same time. For example, higher incidence might reflect greater need and higher mortality may be an outcome of changes in population age structure.

Spatial Distributions

So far we have concentrated on just the first of two aspects of our definition of availability: the total supply of health practitioners and the distribution of that supply. We now turn to the second consideration, geographic concentration or dispersion. A particular locality might have an acceptable level of availability of health care resources in numerical terms, but the spatial location of those resources in relation to the populations being served might be unacceptable according to certain criteria. What we are concerned about here is the distance (measured in various ways) between health care providers and potential clients, or what is often called physical or geographical accessibility. The issue of physical accessibility is especially acute in rural areas where population density may be very low and people may be widely dispersed. Two geographers, Joseph and Phillips (1984) use the term *potential* accessibility to represent physical accessibility to resources as distinct from *revealed* accessibility, which they equate with actual utilization of resources. Joseph and Bantock (1982) suggest that regional accessibility measures be used. In the examples above, we have shown regional availability using physician-to-population ratios; we discuss ways to calculate physical accessibility from this point on.

Measuring physical accessibility. The basic ingredients of measures of physical accessibility are the number of medical resources available within a prescribed travel range of potential consumers and the relative locations of clients and providers. Relative location is measured in terms of map distance, road distance, or travel time. It must also be recognized that the likelihood of patient/provider contact often decreases with increasing distance; this phenomenon is known as distance decay or the friction of distance. The exact nature of the distance decay is usually determined empirically, and the technical approach that should be used is the subject of controversy (i.e., should one use a power or negative exponential function for the distance variable?).

Joseph and Bantock (1982) provide an algebraic approach for measuring physical accessibility to general practitioners (GPs):

$$(1) \quad A_i = \sum_j \frac{GP_j}{d_{ij}^b} \quad \text{where:}$$

$A_{(i)}$ = potential physical accessibility of area i to GPs;

$GP_{(j)}$ = GPs at j within range of area i;

$d_{(ij)}$ = distance between i and j; and

b = exponent on distance.

This formula essentially provides an overall index that describes the number of providers (GPs in this case) who are accessible based on a prescribed standard within a prescribed area, independent of the location of the population within the area. They then modify this equation to take into account the fact that physicians in heavily populated catchment areas are very likely to be less available than those in less densely populated areas. They estimate differential availability using the equation:

$$(2) \quad D_j = \sum_i \frac{P_i}{d_{ji}^b} \quad \text{where:}$$

$D_{(j)}$ = potential demand on a GP at j;

$P_{(i)}$ = population in area i;

and $d_{(ji)}$ and b are as above.

Combining the original equation and the modifying equation produces:

$$(3) \quad A_i^* = \sum_j \left(\frac{GP_j}{\sum_i \dfrac{P_i}{d_{ji}^b}} \Bigg/ d_{ij}^b \right)$$

To illustrate the use of their methods, Joseph and Bantock made a study of Wellington County in southern Ontario, Canada (Figure 5-8). The major urban area is Guelph; several smaller places are scattered throughout the county. Population data were calculated at the level of enumeration areas (EAs) which are the basic areal units for the Canadian Census, and the locations of general practitioners (GPs) came from a local District Health Council survey. Because GPs who lived outside Wellington County served people in the county, they were included in the calculations. Note that 52 of the 89 GPs included in the study were located in Guelph. Distances were measured between centroids of EAs. The exponent on distance, *b*, in equation (3) was set equal to 2, a value shown to give good results in previous empirical work. The exponent estimates the degree to which distance makes a difference in going to a doctor and is a "best guess" parameter in the formula. In order to compare the effect of range on accessibility, range was set at 5, 10, and 15 miles in variants of the analysis. Accessibility indices for the EAs were multiplied by 10,000 for ease of interpretation.

In Figure 5-9a, only physicians within a distance of five miles from populations were included. The map shows a strong contrast in accessibility between EAs close to urban places (where the GPs are) and those that are not close. Several EAs are more than five miles from any GP and so have an accessibility index of 0.0. To produce Figure 5-9b, the range has been extended to 10 miles. Accessibility scores increase over those shown in Figure 5-9a; one EA (interestingly, quite close to Guelph) has a score of 0.0, and disparities among EAs are reduced somewhat. A range of 15 miles (Figure 5-9c) produces a positive accessibility score for all EAs, but little overall change from the 10 mile range, due basically to the effect of the exponent on distance in equation (3).

To demonstrate the impact of including equation (2), which measures physician availability, Joseph and Bantock calculated accessibility indices for EAs using equation (1) at a range of 10 miles (Figure 5-9d). Comparing Figures 5-9b (weighted by physician availability) and 5-9d (unweighted), we see that accessibility scores in the latter are generally lower and the highest unweighted scores are also much more concentrated around Guelph. In Figure 5-9b, rural areas quite far from Guelph have relatively good scores—the point being that "[i]n all probability, although physicians in more isolated rural areas may be at some distance from potential clients, they are likely to be more available to them, which serves to compensate in part for the inherent disadvantage of isolation from major, urban concentrations of general practitioners" (Joseph & Bantock, 1982).

Figure 5-8 **Guelph and Vicinity, Southern Ontario**

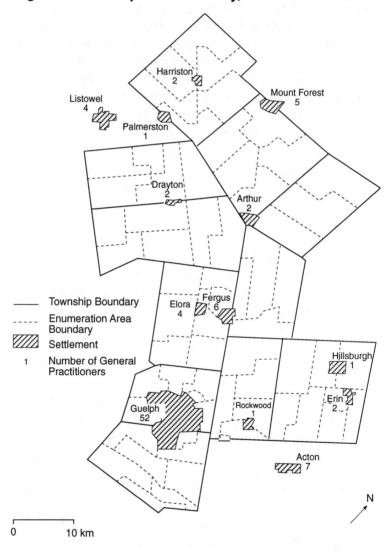

Township Boundary

Enumeration Area
Boundary

Settlement

1 Number of General
Practitioners

0   10 km

N

Source: Adapted from Joseph and Bantock, 1982.
Produced by: NC Rural Health Research Program, Cecil G. Sheps Center for Health
Services Research, UNC - Chapel Hill.

More sophisticated analyses can be performed, for example, a procedure using regression analysis that takes into consideration more factors that might affect use including age and sex categorization. The approach we have outlined above "calculates the potential spatial access of various communities to the medical care delivery system," whereas a regression-based approach "estimates the overall potential effectiveness of the delivery system in overcoming distance barriers" (Thouez, Bodson & Joseph, 1988). This extension of the analysis might be useful in more precisely addressing the distance barriers associated with rural populations. However, its complexity requires much greater computational work and may not be accessible to the non-specialist.

Thresholds for Specialties

One way to look at the spatial component of availability is to estimate the threshold for a medical service and then determine what percentage of the target population falls within that threshold. The threshold might be a certain population size or a certain distance measure. Central Place Theory states that higher order goods and services require higher population thresholds and wider geographic ranges. Gober and Gordon (1980) derived a table of suggested thresholds for several different physician specialties based on the number of practitioners in each category. In their study of Phoenix, Arizona, they used the standard distance measure to show that some types of physicians were more widely dispersed than others throughout the city. In general, primary care physicians, who had the lowest population thresholds, were more widely dispersed (although not to the same extent as the population itself).

Equity Issues

Why Study Equity?

It has been recognized for a long time that the distribution of health care resources in the United States is not equitable across regions based on different geographic scales. Large urban areas tend to attract more resources than do smaller urban places and rural

Figure 5-9
Potential Physical Accessibility to General Practitioners
Guelph and Vicinity, Southern Ontario

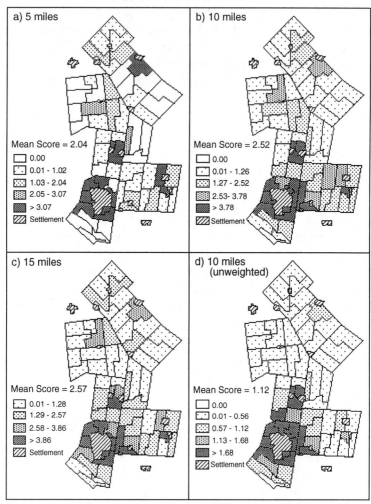

a) 5 miles

Mean Score = 2.04
☐ 0.00
▣ 0.01 - 1.02
▦ 1.03 - 2.04
▩ 2.05 - 3.07
■ > 3.07
▨ Settlement

b) 10 miles

Mean Score = 2.52
☐ 0.00
▣ 0.01 - 1.26
▦ 1.27 - 2.52
▩ 2.53 - 3.78
■ > 3.78
▨ Settlement

c) 15 miles

Mean Score = 2.57
▣ 0.01 - 1.28
▦ 1.29 - 2.57
▩ 2.58 - 3.86
■ > 3.86
▨ Settlement

d) 10 miles
(unweighted)

Mean Score = 1.12
☐ 0.00
▣ 0.01 - 0.56
▦ 0.57 - 1.12
▩ 1.13 - 1.68
■ > 1.68
▨ Settlement

Source: Adapted from Joseph and Bantock, 1982.

areas, but there are often gross inequities within large urban areas. Achieving equity in health care provision is an extremely thorny problem. Most Americans believe that we are endowed with equal rights, which should, in the minds of many, include equal access to health care. Some might say that we should not worry about health care equity, however, as the relationship between health care expenditures and outcomes is weak. For example, in an earlier discussion, the point was made that practitioner-to-population ratios are not necessarily positively correlated with indices of better health. However, the public believes services to be important and desires greater equity in service provision and distribution (Fein, 1972).

Equity Concepts and Measures

How do we measure equity? There are substantially different criteria on which we could base equity: we could say that equity is achieved when different people either a) have equal resources *available* to them for their care, b) *use* equal amounts of assets for care, or c) achieve equal health *outcomes*. We might also distinguish between horizontal and vertical equity. Horizontal equity refers to the provision of the same set of services for people in approximately the same economic circumstances and is essentially an availability question. Vertical equity refers to provision to people of different economic circumstances, or "fairness." Here we deal with horizontal equity when we compare availability among geographic units, but we have also dealt with vertical equity in our discussion of availability for different population subgroups.

There are two basic approaches to equity that we, as a nation or society, could take. One is to attempt to make health care available or accessible on a financially equitable basis. To determine the degree to which we meet this goal would require examination of payment schemes, insurance schemes, and government programs such as Medicare and Medicaid. The second approach is to guarantee equal availability of resources, especially providers. This is the prevailing view of equity in the US and to measure it we must examine the distribution of our resources. We have considered only one aspect of this system, the distribution of resources. This view of equity is limited but makes comparisons more tractable.

In the introduction to this chapter, we alluded to some of the factors behind resource distributions. Fein (1972) states that availability of physicians (which he takes to be the core of the health care system) depends on two main factors, specialization and location. The proportion of physicians trained and practicing as specialists continues to increase, some say to the great detriment of the nation's health (COGME, 1992). Since specialists require relatively large threshold populations, they tend to locate in larger and more densely populated areas. In addition, most physicians are relatively free to locate where they find conditions suitable to their needs and desires, without paying a great deal of attention to consumer demand or worrying much about government regulations (there are exceptions: a few physicians, for example, are fulfilling pay-back obligations to the federal government through the National Health Services Corps (NHSC) and are located in places for short tenures). We can measure the *result* of this freedom of movement and the tendency toward specialization, but measurement does not solve the problem although it may suggest ways of changing the process itself, or of identifying high-risk areas where government intervention might be most useful.

Scale at Which Equity is Measured

The question of what geographic scale is the best one to use in measuring equity arises, just as it did for availability. State planners might be concerned that several regions within the state (e.g., AHECs) have more or less equal oncology provider-to-population ratios. Some county health officials, on the other hand, might complain that they are poorly served when compared with neighboring counties. To address this problem, we refer back to our discussion of the importance of scale with regard to physician specialty and the population threshold required for viable practices. If, for example, the threshold for an oncology specialty encompasses several counties, then county comparisons make little sense, while comparisons among clusters of counties would be useful.

Equity and Regionalization

There is a connection between the problems of how to achieve equity and how to develop the most efficacious regionalization of health care provision. Assuming that a reasonable geographic scale for analyzing equity has been agreed upon, policies could target both the structures of regions as well as the distribution of resources within regions. Regions would be created that had equal supplies of resources rather than an inter-regional disparity. At the same time resources would be re-distributed within regions to equalize intra-region access.

Measuring Inequality

Several measures of assessing inequality in the geographic distribution of health manpower are available. These include concentration ratios, location quotients, the coefficient of localization, and Gini coefficients which are used in conjunction with the Lorenz curve.

One of the most common measures used in the medical geography literature is the *location quotient*. The location quotient (LQ) is an index for comparing an area's share of a particular activity with the area's share of some basic characteristic, usually population or area. (See Chapter 3 for a more extensive discussion of location quotients.)

For our purposes, we are looking at the share of physicians in a particular county or AHEC area compared to a correspondingly larger area's share of physicians. Figures 5-10 through 5-12 use location quotients to look at the distribution of core (or primary care) physicians in North Carolina. Core physician specialties are those necessary to sustain a primary medical care system in a community. Figure 5-10 depicts location quotients at a county scale relative to the overall presence of core physicians in the State. A location quotient of 1.0 (or close to unity, in this case between 0.7 and 1.1) reflects an area whose share of physicians is in accordance with that of the larger base area (county vs. state). When LQ > 1, there is a higher concentration of physicians relative to the base; LQ < 1 indicates that the area has a lower concentration of physicians

Figure 5-10 **Core Physicians, Location Quotients for Counties, 1990**

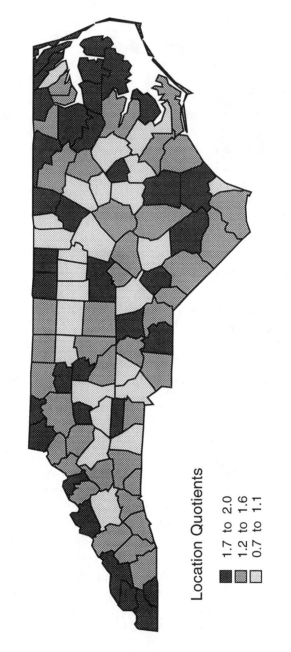

Location Quotients

■ 1.7 to 2.0
▨ 1.2 to 1.6
▢ 0.7 to 1.1

Data Source: 1990 NC Board of Medical Examiners Licensing Data, maintained by the Cecil G. Sheps Center for Health Services Research.
Produced by: NC Rural Health Research Program, Cecil G. Sheps Center for Health Services Research, UNC - Chapel Hill.

Figure 5-11 **Core Physicians, Location Quotients for AHEC Regions, 1990**

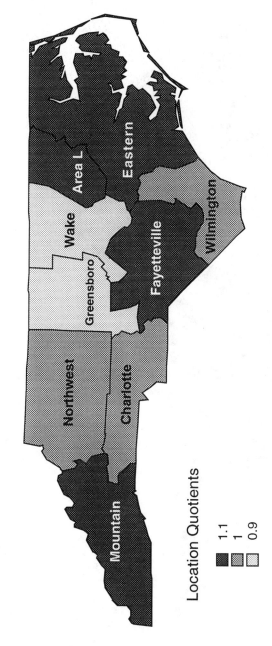

Location Quotients

■ 1.1
▨ 1
▨ 0.9

Data Source: 1990 NC Board of Medical Examiners Licensing Data, maintained by the Cecil G. Sheps Center for Health Services Research.
Produced by: NC Rural Health Research Program, Cecil G. Sheps Center for Health Services Research, UNC - Chapel Hill.

Figure 5-12   **Core Physicians, Location Quotients for Counties within AHEC Regions, 1990**

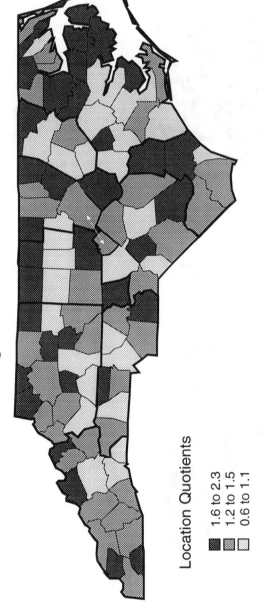

Location Quotients

- 1.6 to 2.3
- 1.2 to 1.5
- 0.6 to 1.1

Data Source: 1990 NC Board of Medical Examiners Licensing Data, maintained by the Cecil G. Sheps Center for Health Services Research.
Produced by: NC Rural Health Research Program, Cecil G. Sheps Center for Health Services Research, UNC - Chapel Hill.

than the base area. Certain inequities are obvious, but we've already noted with oncologists that examination at a smaller scale may be more useful. Figure 5-11 depicts location quotients by AHEC regions. At this scale, very little discrepancy exists. It is only when you analyze intra-AHEC area variation that inequalities become apparent. This is most pronounced for the Eastern AHEC in Figure 5-12.

Location quotients are fairly simple to compute with readily available data and in that sense are useful (see Chapter 3). Isard and Moses (1960) caution, however, that the information provided— that one region has more or less than its proportionate share of something (in this case physicians)—does not necessarily tell us much. They suggest that this measure is most useful in exploratory, hypothesis-generating research. The other major disadvantage relates to the chosen scale of analysis where a large number of areas (e.g., census tracts in an urban area) generates a large number of LQs. This can be a rather inefficient form of summary even when mapped. The Coefficient of Localization has been suggested as a preferable alternative in terms of data summary. Joseph (1982) provides a succinct and easy to follow discussion of its interpretation.

The *Gini coefficient* is the index most commonly used in describing inequality in the distribution of a resource. Corrado Gini proposed this index in 1912 to measure the distribution of incomes. It has since been adapted to other uses including the area of medical resources to illustrate distributions of discrete units such as health personnel. The calculation of the Gini index has been modified over time and computational variations have been proposed to improve the accuracy and applicability of summary measures of inequality. This reflects Gini's use of two indices, the Mean Relative Difference and the Coefficient of Inequality. The Gini coefficient described here can be explained best in the context of the Lorenz curve, which is a graphical representation of the distribution of a resource.

Similar to location quotients, the Lorenz curve compares the areal distribution of an activity to its base distribution. A distribution of resources may be depicted as a curve, the Lorenz curve, which shows the cumulative supply of a particular resource. If the activity is evenly distributed across areas in a region, then the Lorenz curve is a straight line following a 45-degree angle from the origin. The Lorenz curve is created after the holdings in a population are ordered from those with the least to those with the most. The cumulative proportion of those with the least is reflected by the slope of the line in the lower left hand corner. For a large degree of concentration, the line starts out very flat and then begins to rise at a higher rate until it is almost vertical toward the right hand side of a graph plotting the curve. The more concentrated an activity is, the further the Lorenz curve deviates from the diagonal. This technique provides a graphical summary of the degree of inequality that is easy to comprehend.

Figure 5-13 presents the Lorenz curve for the core (primary care) physician distribution in the Fayetteville AHEC, one of the nine regions in North Carolina assigned to a regional Area Health Education Center. The curve below the 45-degree line of equality represents the actual distribution of physicians based on county aggregates. The Gini index essentially measures the area between the actual and the ideal distribution, that is, the 45-degree line and the curve plotted by the cumulative proportion of physicians against the cumulative proportion of population. This is an alternative depiction of the intra-AHEC variation in the availability of core physicians depicted in Figure 5-12 as a choroplethic map that describes deviations from the mean distribution. Lorenz curves which plot the actual distribution of physicians against population could be plotted for any physician specialty.

One means of construction is a geometric method in which discrete points are plotted and connected to form the Lorenz curve. The method follows these steps:

1. Calculate the location quotients for the various areas in a region.

2. Reorder the areas in decreasing order of their location quotients.

Figure 5-13
Lorenz Curve for Core Physician Distribution,
Fayetteville AHEC, October 1990

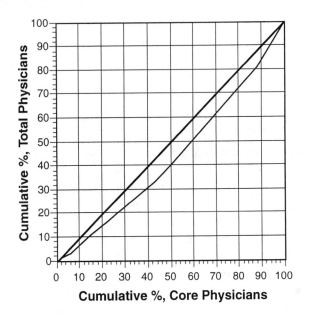

3. Cumulate the percentage distributions of both the activity and the base in the order determined in the previous ranking.

4. Graph the cumulated percentages for the activity and the base and join them to form the Lorenz curve.

Smaller values of the Gini coefficient indicate similarity between the areal distribution of the base and the activity. As they increase, the similarity between the base and the activity decreases. Another index of inequality, the Index of Dissimilarity, perfected by Otis and Beverly Duncan (1955), is also used to compare distributional differences between groups. Its classic use has been in the comparison of population characteristics of communities or regions.

The strengths and weaknesses of the various ways to calculate the Gini index and the specifics of index construction are discussed in depth by Philip Coulter in his book, *Measuring Inequality: A Methodological Handbook* (1989). James Morrow (1979) used the Gini index to assess changes in physician distribution in the United States in an early use of the index to evaluate the geographic distribution of health manpower and identify certain inequalities. It is important to note that the Gini index can create equal summary values for very different distributions and, before it is used, the implications of its applicability to a particular distribution should be carefully considered.

We have attempted to provide a discussion of some of the more useful tools and techniques used in evaluating the distribution of health professionals. We have focused our examples on physicians but recognize the existence of many different types of health professionals—each with unique concerns and characteristics pertinent to the evaluation of their distribution. The techniques presented here can be generally applied to any of these groups. As always, however, any study of health professional distribution is only as valid as the underlying quality of the available data.

▷ P O I N T
▷ OF DEPARTURE

Community-Based Measures
of Underservice
Thomas C. Ricketts

The problem of shortages of health professionals, especially physicians, in communities in the United States is a longstanding one. Aggregate measures of physician supply and need have attracted national attention from time to time—witness the degree of concern and the amount of comment that accompanied the reports by the Graduate Medical Education National Advisory Committee (GMENAC) in the 1980's, and, to a lesser extent the Council on Graduate Medical Education (COGME) in this decade. The need for a provider is more sharply felt by local, and especially rural, communities where the name of a doctor who left or passed away is known to all and the dilemma of a shortage is personal. Programs to meet the needs of these communities were idiosyncratic and equally personal before the federal government recognized health professional shortages as a national problem and the Congress began to appropriate money to fill the needs. Funding the National Health Service Corps and the Neighborhood Health Centers programs meant that methods had to be put in place to identify priority communities where the shortages were most severe. These changes shifted the focus from isolated, previously self-sufficient areas to a more global perspective of health care manpower need (see Figure 5-14).

P
O
I
N
T

O
F

D
E
P
A
R
T
U
R
E

To determine whether or not a community has a provider shortage, agencies have set criteria that are often neither directly derived from nor linked to aggregate approaches like those developed by the GMENAC. In the development of indicators of need, there were two federal approaches for the identification of areas to which programs were to be targeted: the Critical Health Manpower (now Professional) Shortage Area Criteria, and the Index of Medical Underservice used to identify Medically Underserved Areas. The former were used for National Health Service Corps placements, and the latter originally for targeting locations for the development of HMOs and later for qualification of a site for Bureau of Community Health Services (BCHS)[1] programs including Community and Migrant Health Centers (Lee, 1979).

The construction of needs standards for communities required the delineation of a service area or boundary for the geographic units to be designated. The original 1965 loan cancellation legislation from the US Congress, which initiated federal involvement in addressing shortages, gave no guidance for this determination. However, since data were readily available for counties, these became the basic unit of designation and a set of "Health Manpower Shortage Areas" was published in the *Federal Register* in February of 1974. During the development of the National Health Service Corps regulations there was some concern that the designation process focused too much on "manpower" rather than "health service scarcity of all types" (Health Services Administration, 1973). The Health Scarcity Area Identification Program was meant to centralize the process of designations for all of the programs in the Department of Health, Education and Welfare that depended upon identification of a shortage area. The program

[1] BCHS later became the Bureau of Health Care Delivery and Assistance (BHCDA), then the Bureau of Primary Health Care (BPHC).

Figure 5-14 **North Carolina Active, Non-Federal Primary Care Physicians Changes in Numbers by County, 1985-1990**

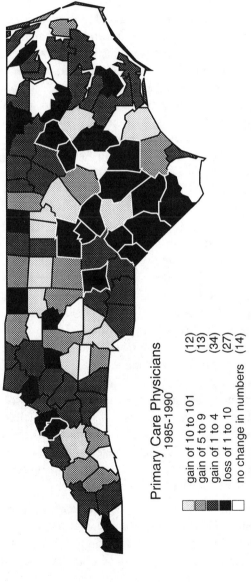

Primary Care Physicians
1985-1990

gain of 10 to 101	(12)
gain of 5 to 9	(13)
gain of 1 to 4	(34)
loss of 1 to 10	(27)
no change in numbers	(14)

Data Source: NC Board of Medical Examiners Data Files; maintained by the Cecil G. Sheps Center for Health Services Research, UNC - Chapel Hill.
Produced by: NC Rural Health Research Program, UNC - Chapel Hill.

P
O
I
N
T

O
F

D
E
P
A
R
T
U
R
E

was also to develop a Master Health Service Scarcity Area Database. The program eventually identified 1,333 areas as of December 31, 1972. The basis for designation was a complex set of criteria that passed through multiple levels of state and federal agencies; several key characteristics of the designation process were institutionalized in the process: 1) the areas could be Census tracts, minor civil divisions, or full counties; 2) there were "special criteria that took into consideration travel times and special population groups"; 3) access barriers are considered; and 4) the process would consider a broad range of professions and services. The process would identify "factors leading to or causing the shortage ... which helps to amplify the stated health service needs of the area" (HSA, 1973). The Health Service Scarcity idea did not move far beyond the Bureau of Community Health Services, and when a listing of areas was published in the *Federal Register* they appeared as Critical Health Manpower Shortage Areas (CMHSAs), which are different from the HMSAs described above. The criterion for designation as a physician shortage area was a population-to-provider ratio of 4,000:1 and this figure was based upon the distribution of population-to-provider ratios for all US counties. It was felt that counties falling in the bottom quartile were "underserved" or had a "shortage" and the cutoff for the bottom quartile at that time was the 4,000:1 level. The actual designation of areas involved the comprehensive health planning agencies in each state and was done on a state-by-state basis with the result that, as of September 30, 1977, approximately 770 US counties and 400 subcounty areas were designated as critical medical shortage areas. The great majority of these areas were rural.

The Nurse Training Act of 1971 called for the establishment of nursing shortage areas where nurses could have their loan obligations excused through service. The designations were based on ratios of optimal-to-actual nurse staffing for health care facilities in each county after the idea of using a nurse-to-population ratio was rejected. A listing of 541 nursing shortage counties, 18 percent of the national total, was published in June, 1976.

The Health Maintenance Organization Act of 1973 introduced the concept of a "medically underserved area" and its subsequent definition was based on an index developed by the Health Services Research Group at the University of Wisconsin (1975). The development of that index proceeded in a very comprehensive and painstaking manner as consultants reviewed 72 different variables to find a reasonable reduced set which would allow the research team to predict with accuracy counties, towns, cities and groups of census tracts that were, in the independent opinion of experts, underserved (Kushman, 1977; Wysong, 1975; Kleinman & Wilson, 1977). Four variables were selected: 1) the percentage of persons in poverty, 2) the percentage of the population over the age of 65, 3) the infant mortality rate, and 4) the number of primary care physicians per 1,000 population. A listing of Medically Underserved Areas (MUAs) was published in the *Federal Register* in September 1975, updated in 1976, and the final full list published in 1981. Since that date only individual notifications of designations or withdrawals of designations have been published.

The passage of the Health Professions Educational Assistance Act of 1976 (PL 94-484) called for a whole new set of regulations concerning the designation of health manpower shortage areas. The designation process was divided into seven categories: 1) primary medical care manpower, including physician assistants and nurse practitioners; 2) dental manpower including auxiliaries; 3) psychiatric manpower, including related therapeutic practitioners; 4) vision care manpower, optometrists and ophthalmologists; 5) podiatric manpower; 6) pharmacy manpower; and 7) veterinary manpower. The process of

POINT OF DEPARTURE

designation was intended to make it easier to recognize urban as well as rural shortage areas by allowing for the identification of population subgroups whose needs might be measured in ways other than through provider-to-population ratios. The definition of the areas to be designated revolved around the idea of a "rational service area" that was roughly described by a travel time of 30 minutes for primary medical care and 40 minutes for dental care in rural areas. The areas were also to be "contiguous" but the notion of identified special populations made the application of this concept somewhat inconsistent with a strict definition of contiguous. The basic population-to-provider ratio for primary care manpower was set at 3,500-to-1 as this represented 150 percent of the median ratio for all US counties and, again, qualified approximately the bottom quartile of US counties for initial designation. The actual designation process involved local and state planning agencies and interested groups, including medical societies and civic organizations involved in the planning process. These review processes were later relaxed as the regulations were revised to overrule local medical and dental associations that were commonly objecting to designations and placements of National Health Service Corps personnel.

The shortage area criteria that were developed prior to 1980 were the subject of two major reviews and evaluations. The first, completed by Mathematica Policy Research for the US Bureau of Health Professions (1980), reviewed the criteria for designation, relevant literature, and comments on the regulations as published in 1978 and summarized the process of designation. The report suggested several changes to the criteria and the process but did not propose any fundamental changes to the assumptions behind them. The second evaluation compared the CHMSA criteria for designation to four other approaches: the Index of Medical Underservice, the Utilization Deficit Index, the Deaths Averted Index, and the Use/Need Index (US Bureau of Health Professions, 1983). The alternatives did not appear to be superior in their sensitivity and they generally identified similar groups of counties and areas.

The Bureau of Health Care Delivery and Assistance (now BPHC) has attempted to streamline the designation process and make it understandable to potential designees and state officials through workshops and by funding several regionally based organizations that provide technical assistance to communities, state agencies, and professionals. The designation process is a very important step in the acquisition of resources for underserved communities and the regulations can potentially cost individual communities substantially as a result of small adjustments in the rules. The process is somewhat flexible and it is anticipated that more "population groups" including indigents and minority populations will be designated in the future (Nutting, 1987). The sensitivity of the formula and its centrality to the politics of programmatic activity for rural communities was demonstrated in late 1989 when the Department of Health and Human Services proposed modifying the process to exclude from eligibility for a National Health Service Corps placement HMSAs that might require less than a full-time provider (Shortage area criteria, 1989). It was expected that this change would reduce the number of rural primary care HMSAs from 1,337 to 817 (NRHA helps defeat proposed rule, 1989); this rule change was not adapted.

The designation process for Critical Health Manpower Shortage Areas, now Critical Health Professional Shortage Areas, remains essentially the same process as that developed under the direction of the Health Professions Educational Assistance Act of 1976, with the burden for identification of new CHPSAs placed on the states, who must apply to the US Division of Shortage Designation in the Bureau of Primary Health Care. Areas designated for three continuous years are dropped from designation unless the state involved produces more current evidence to continue the designation. The designations are reviewed and published in the *Federal Register* from time to time. The most recent designation list, current through September 30, 1993, listed a total 2,448 medical care shortage places with a total population of 42,787,156 and a need for 4,559 practitioners to remove that total designation (US Division of Shortage Designation, 1993).

▷ P O I N T
▷ OF DEPARTURE

Tracking Doctors Into
the Twenty-First Century
Thomas R. Konrad

To evaluate efforts at physician workforce reform being initiated by health care policy makers, we need longitudinal studies of physicians' specialty choice and practice location. Sound policy in this area requires a solid database for measuring physician migration and related shifts in practice settings and specialties. Despite these needs, much of the research done to date about the movement of physicians has relied on inferences from cross-sectional studies of physician distribution by specialty and practice location.

Such studies compare measures of physician availability (e.g., physician-to-population ratios) across regions or states, or among different types of communities (e.g., urban, suburban, rural). When these types of measures are examined at different times and ratios are observed as increasing or decreasing, conclusions are often drawn about whether or not availability of physicians to a population is "improving" or "worsening." Occasionally, a series of cross-sectional studies is examined to assess whether or not physicians are "going to" or "leaving" certain areas. Considerable portions of the academic and policy literature and federal regulations are based on such studies. Prominent examples of this approach are the so-called "RAND" studies of the early 1980's (Williams et al., 1983; Newhouse et al., 1982a,b,c). From a geographic perspective, however, such an approach has had a distinct limitation—despite inferences drawn about migration, the approach is static rather than dynamic.

Every year about 16,000 new physicians enter the workforce and, at the same time, an unknown but probably smaller number of physicians leaves the work force temporarily or permanently through death, disability, limited periods of inactivity, changes to a non-medical career, or retirement. In addition to these changes in overall supply, physicians exhibit geographic mobility linked to changes in the type and/or location of their practices. Because the total number of physicians in the US exceeds 600,000, change in the overall supply and distribution of physicians occurs slowly. Thus even if global interventions aimed at influencing the supply and distribution of physicians were extraordinarily effective in reaching their intended targets, it would take a long time for these effects to be reflected in the overall physician population.

This "persistence of aggregates" phenomenon means, for example, that the effects of decisions made today to "correct" specialty distribution by altering the mix of residency training slots will not really be felt until the third decade of the twenty-first century (Kindig & Movassaghi, 1989; COGME, 1992). The apparent inertia in the supply and distribution of physicians occurs despite the fact that dramatic changes may be unfolding rapidly when specific cohorts, sectors, or localities are examined. Such a situation has led policy analysts to search for more sensitive indicators of the impact of various educational and financing policies aimed at affecting physician distribution, in terms of both practice content and location. Not surprisingly, just as economists tend to focus their attention on what happens "at the margin," policy analysts find it useful to focus their attention on more proximate indicators of supply. These include not only "enters" and "exits" from the stock of physicians, but also those transitions associated with job mobility and geographic relocation. Examples of this more recent dynamic approach can be found in studies focusing on national (Wright, 1985; Madison & Combs, 1981) or regional data sets (Kindig et al., 1992; Horner et al., 1993), or smaller samples of physicians (Pathman et al., 1992; Barnett, 1987,1992).

The primary source of data for many of these studies has been the Physician Masterfile of the American Medical Association. This is the largest and most accurate national roster of physicians in the US. It is continuously updated and periodically archived using a variety of sources, but ultimately relies on elicited self-report. Existing assessments of the quality of the Masterfile as a data source confirm that it is a remarkably good source for the purpose of static analyses (Loft & Ryan, 1985). However, little research has been done upon which to base an assessment of the utility and reliability of dynamic analyses using AMA data. It stands to reason, however, that a physician data source that relies on physicians' self-reports and official records of various sorts in order to determine changes in physician status will contain certain systematic biases in accuracy and coverage. Unfortunately, the greatest inaccuracies are likely to occur precisely at those points of transition which constitute the focus of interest in longitudinal studies. Such personal and professional transitions include the passage from residency to practice, the onset of retirement, migration from one community to another, and the temporary withdrawal from the labor force associated with starting a family.

Although fewer than half of the physicians in the US actually belong to the AMA, the Masterfile aims to be comprehensive in its coverage and very nearly accomplishes this. One of the primary ways in which this is done is the use of a single unique and permanent physician identification number in which are embedded the medical school from which the physician graduated and year of graduation from medical school. This identification number allows tracking of physicians across geographic, career, and personal transitions (e.g., name changes associated with marriage) and is used to help minimize the occurrence of multiple listings of the same physician who might be licensed in more than one state.

Certain core data items on the AMA Masterfile are important in assessing physician career and geographic mobility. These data items may be thought of as being of two types: fixed and variable. Fixed items are those that are unlikely to change over the course of a physician's career; they are helpful in tracking physicians who may have changed their names or in discriminating among physicians with similar names. In addition to the items embedded in the physician's ID number (medical school and year of graduation), fixed items include things such as a physician's first name, gender, and birth year. Several other items are important but variable, or mutable, indicators of the extent or kind of employment or professional role that a physician might be performing. These include the address of the physician, the type of practice and the major professional activity in which he or she is currently engaged, as well as whether the physician is federally employed.

Location data in the AMA Masterfile are based on responses supplied by physicians to a questionnaire called the Record of Physicians' Professional Activities (also known as the PPA questionnaire), which is sent to them by the AMA. "Every four years the PPA questionnaire is mailed to all physicians residing in the US. Between Census years, an elaborate computerized system continually monitors Masterfile data in order to identify and mail questionnaires to physicians who may have had significant changes in their professional activities" (Kletke et al., 1987). Physicians can list a "preferred professional mailing address" on the PPA questionnaire, but if that preferred address is not their "primary office" address, then they are requested to list their "primary office address."

Transition tracking is done by means of the physician questionnaire and is activated as part of the AMA's physician monitoring system. Physicians' names and selected biographical data are entered into the system upon graduation from a US allopathic medical school, using medical student data collected in tandem with the Association of American Medical Colleges. Other nonstandard mechanisms for entry into the system (for foreign medical graduates and "fifth pathway" individuals who did not graduate from medical schools identified by the AMA) come at the time of licensure in one of the several US jurisdictions, based on data sharing agreements with boards of medical examiners in those jurisdictions. For US-trained osteopathic physicians (DOs), enrollment in an AMA-approved residency program may serve as an entry point into the system. An estimated 50 percent of DOs are included on the Masterfile.

Subsequent changes in physician status or location are captured through what might be characterized as "elicited self report." The PPA questionnaire is sent to physicians when the Physician Data Services staff of the AMA suspect a change of address or a change of status to have occurred. Physician responses are then used to update computerized physician records in the system.

Both reactive and proactive evidence trigger these efforts to update the data and arise from a wide array of potential sources. Such an ensemble of techniques for monitoring an occupational group is probably without parallel in the US. The system is, however, differentially effective in determining the extent and timing of physicians' geographic and status mobility since some physicians are more likely to participate than others. Also, individual items on the Physician Masterfile are likely to be updated with differential frequency. Changes in mailing addresses are more likely to trigger a PPA than are changes in practice or principal activity. For this reason, the actual status of "retired" physicians is somewhat problematic at any given time unless this transition occurs along with a geographic move. Shifts in the "preferred office" address can also lead one to believe that a move has taken place, when in fact it has not.

Finding physicians and tracking them involves examining different types of phenomena. We must not only know where they are now, but where they came from. Effective longitudinal monitoring also requires anticipation of where (and when) they might be going to different jobs or locations. Recent developments in the career structure and demographics of the American physician population make the issue of geographic mobility more salient because physicians may be behaving differently than in the past.

This discussion highlights only a select set of the factors that need to be considered when evaluating the issue of physician distribution. Ironically, many of these relatively recent transitions in health professions supply have not only made it more difficult to track physician migration, but have also increased the uncertainty surrounding the question of whether current patterns reflect temporary trends or have long-term implications. In the coming era of health reform we may expect increasing attempts to tackle this issue. Geographic techniques can be a useful tool in improving systems of tracking health professionals and making accurate projections of their supply.

Chapter 6

Regionalization of Health Care

Points of Departure:
Rural Places and Regionalization
Geographic Information Systems (GIS)

Regionalization is an important component of the organization of medical care and is becoming more important as the system moves into a period of rapid change and reform. This chapter examines regionalization as a concept, outlines the history of recent attempts to regionalize, and describes methods to draw regional boundaries and analyze regional systems. We explore the relationship between regions and scale of analysis, indicators of need, the distribution of resources, and the relationship of transportation and movement to regional structures.

The Concept of Regionalization

Regionalization in Geography

A region can be simply defined as a portion of the earth's surface that for some reason is different from the rest of the earth's surface. A region defined in this way is very much a mental construct. One person may choose to divide an area into one set of regions; another may regionalize the same area in a different way. In part, this may be due to different goals, different reasons for subdividing the area. The district sales manager who wishes to determine the precise borders of the sales regions of the company's sales staff would likely create a pattern quite unlike that of a botanist interested in regional variation in tree types. One set of geographers, when subdividing the United States into regions, may well create a map noticeably different from that formed by a second group of geographers simply because they identified different elements as most influential in their patterns.

These varying reasons for regionalizing and different attitudes on the part of regionalizers can obviously lead to the creation of many different maps of an area. None is necessarily any "better" than the others. If it meets the requirements of its creators, if those requirements were reasonably thought out, and if the map is correctly and factually executed, then the regionalization is acceptable. For the geographer, the region can be thought of as a neat system of categorization that allows us to reduce variance for some characteristic or to circumscribe patterns of movement. The goal is to organize that variation into patterns that are perhaps easier to comprehend and useful in recognizing the underlying processes. As with any categorization, the regions are sensible if they succeed in identifying understandable patterns in the facts.

Although regions are traditionally a central theme in geographical writing, geographers have always been reticent about the ways in which regions can be built. Regions can be described in general ways; these usually reflect the areal patterns of human activity. To the geographer, a region can be either nodal or uniform, and it can be single or multifeatured. A *nodal region* (sometimes referred to as a functional region) is identified by a focus (or node), or perhaps multiple foci, and a surrounding area connected to the focus by lines of communication or transportation. The service area of a hospital, with its patient population connected to the hospital by their routes of travel, is an example of a nodal region—as is the area in which people patronize a certain shopping mall or are loyal to a particular baseball team. Such an area might be internally very diverse in appearance with only the one movement pattern tying it together into a region. In comparison, a *uniform region* is assumed to be internally, at least, homogeneous throughout in reference to one or more select variables. The area where a particular species of vegetation is found or that portion of the country where grits remain an acceptable part of breakfast are examples of uniform regions. A *single region* is one that is described by a single characteristic such as ethnicity or income while a *multifeatured region* uses a variety of indicators to identify boundaries.

Regionalization in Health Care

In the broadest sense, regionalization of health care implies an allocation of service delivery or utilization based on geography. Regionalization systems need not be based solely on geography—they can be based on consciously developed markets; the Kaiser-Permanente Medical Care Program is the classic example. While that distinction is important, all health care regionalizations contain some geographic base. Kaiser-Permanente has slowly expanded from the West Coast into other regions based largely on market considerations, but as they expand they identify regions within which centrally located providers can efficiently serve population concentrations.

Such a regionalization may represent identification of existing, but uncontrolled service area boundaries. Setting these regional boundaries may allow a program or company to analyze service utilization. Alternatively, a physician locating a new practice might use such an effort to identify areas that may currently be poorly served. An example of such a regionalization would be a study of the geographic pattern of hospital utilization drawn from a patient origin survey.

More recently, health care regionalizations have usually taken the form of a "rationalization," where the goal is to "... alter the functions of—and the relationships between—health providers within an area in order to achieve better access to health care, a higher quality of service, lower costs, greater equity, and more responsiveness to consumer needs and desires" (Ginzberg, 1977). Arguments for such an approach have usually centered upon either cost reduction— "... savings would accrue by using centralized facilities at fewer hospitals with high patient volumes, rather than by offering specialized services at every medical center regardless of utilization" (Finkler, 1979)—or an improvement in quality of care. A number of studies over the past few years have documented a correlation between low volumes of patients in a hospital who have a particular procedure or diagnosis and the number of subsequent deaths or complications (Maerki, Luft & Hunt, 1986). These arguments for centralization and concentration can be countered by their concomitant reductions in access and the fact that not all conditions can be treated efficiently or effectively at higher volumes.

Efforts to regionalize (i.e., rationalize) health care in the United States usually follow one or more of three approaches: through patient flow, the allocation of health facilities, or the location of health manpower. All such efforts are strongly influenced by the pluralism of the health industry. Private health insurance, consumers, and the federal government provide most health payments. Authority over regulation, licensing, and certification of health services is provided for at the state level. Professional organizations, usually operating at the state or local level, often have a major impact on the decision-making process. Thus, no one group dominates the country's health delivery system. Organized interest groups and the federal government have been most important in shaping a health care delivery system on which unorganized customers have had little impact.

Therefore, Two Meanings of "Regionalization"

There are distinct differences between the meaning the geographer usually gives to the term regionalization and its current, implied definition in health care delivery studies. The distinction is an important one. As used by the geographer, it simply means the process of creating regions, whatever their nature. To the health care professional or planner, the term usually means a hierarchy of services in a system where participating elements create organized programs to provide care at given levels of quality or intensity within designated geographic areas, perhaps dictating interrelationships for consultation and referral to maximize the effectiveness of the system while attempting to limit cost.

We suggest here that both definitions, both uses, have meaning for health care. While much of the remaining discussion will focus upon the current health care definition, the geographer's perspective provides the opportunity to ask, and answer, other useful questions.

A History of Health Care Regionalization in the United States

There has been less concern about hierarchical regionalization of health care here in the United States than in most other developed countries. The capitalist system often encourages competition among resources and can, therefore, tend to discourage efforts at rationalization. Still, there have been at least ten broad attempts to regionalize aspects of this country's delivery system. For example:

- Local attempts aimed at the regionalization of American health care predate World War II. The first may have been the voluntary organization, initially funded by the Bingham Associates Fund, to lessen the isolation of rural physicians in Maine in the 1930's. A hierarchical system was encouraged, with hospitals in Lewiston and Bangor each affiliated with perhaps ten community hospitals.

- Also in the 1930's, the city of New York, concerned over health care costs during the Depression, issued a lengthy *Hospital Survey of New York* that suggested, among other things, a single agency to monitor both public and private hospitals and if necessary develop suggestions for action to lower costs.

- The Roosevelt Administration proposed construction of a series of rural hospitals late in the decade based on regional principles—an action that was roundly opposed by the American Hospital Association.

Hill-Burton Act

The Hill-Burton Act, or more precisely the Hospital Survey and Construction Act of 1946, formed the basis of the first national program of health care regionalization. The Act gave federal support to states for hospital construction with each state responsible for inventorying its own need and creating an acceptable plan for use of the funds. Hospitals serving rural areas were at first given priority, although amendments to the Act gradually shifted priority to urban areas.

Each state was obliged to identify general hospital service areas or functional service boundaries as part of its plan. In the great majority of cases, boundaries were placed along existing county borders. Political complexities plus a common lack of more detailed service area information discouraged deviation away from this county boundary orientation.

The Public Health Service Act

The Hill-Burton Act was actually an act to amend the Public Health Service Act of 1944. That Act was designed to bring together in one statute all legislation concerning the Public Health Service (PHS). As part of the initial activities of the newly constituted PHS, the Surgeon General in 1945 released a map of health service areas in the United States (Figure 6-1). The areas were based on the pattern of existing hospital facilities. All boundaries followed county lines and none crossed state borders. Although of limited importance in planning implementation, this was the first formal, federal attempt to define service areas at the national level.

American Medical Association
Medical Service Areas

In the late 1940's, the American Medical Association (AMA) offered its own identification of US medical service areas (Figure

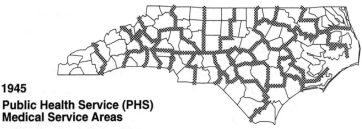

1945

**Public Health Service (PHS)
Medical Service Areas**

- Followed county and state boundaries
- Identified four types of medical service areas—primary, secondary, proposed secondary and isolated—according to existing facilities

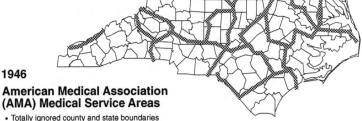

1946

**American Medical Association
(AMA) Medical Service Areas**

- Totally ignored county and state boundaries
- Identified geographic trade areas for physician services

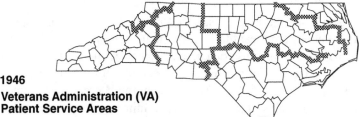

1946

**Veterans Administration (VA)
Patient Service Areas**

- Totally ignored county and state boundaries
- Changed boundaries to accomodate shifting patient origin areas
- Emphasized geographic efficiency of boundaries with maximum availability to services and regional efficency as well as minimum patient travel time and cost

Sources: Florin, 1980. In: *Conceptual and Methodological Issues in Medical Geography*, and Whittington, 1992. Veterans Administration, personal communication.

Figure 6-1 **Health Service Area Regionalization Plans
Developed Under Categorical Grants**

6-1). The AMA used a trading area concept—the geographic trade areas for physicians in communities of different size. At the lower end were some 16,000 secondary medical centers (places with at least one physician). Of greater importance were 964 primary centers (places that were a primary source of care for a surrounding area) and 88 prime-primary centers (places that provided every type of medical care).

The AMA map was dramatically unlike the earlier PHS Medical Service Area map. Most state and county boundaries were completely ignored. What was instead created was a series of nodal regions. The three-tiered arrangement implied a hierarchical orientation, although no such differentiation was made on the AMA map.

Veterans Administration Medical Care Program

The Veterans Administration (VA) system of health care delivery is the clearest example of a national US system implemented and administered through a regional model (Figure 6-1). The entire VA system, including over 150 hospitals and some 200 clinics and nursing homes, is administered through a central headquarters and a number of regional offices. Each region includes several hospital districts within which hospitals are organized to share equipment and services. Patients normally use the nearest hospital, but may be sent to another facility for specialized care.

The VA hospital districts, and especially the individual hospital service areas, are meant to identify natural service areas for each hospital. Patterns of use do change, however, and the boundaries are periodically redefined to compensate for these shifts. Boundaries generally follow county borders but freely cross state boundaries. The overall system, designed to minimize cost and maximize availability, is strongly hierarchical and prescriptive for the system. Participants are required to respect boundaries for planning and allocation but patients can still choose to go to a hospital other than the one closest to them.

Comprehensive Health Planning Areas

The Public Health Service Act of 1944 was modified in 1966 to provide for more efficient use of federal funds for planning and support

Block Grants

Characteristics of these plans included:
- Generally followed county and state political boundaries

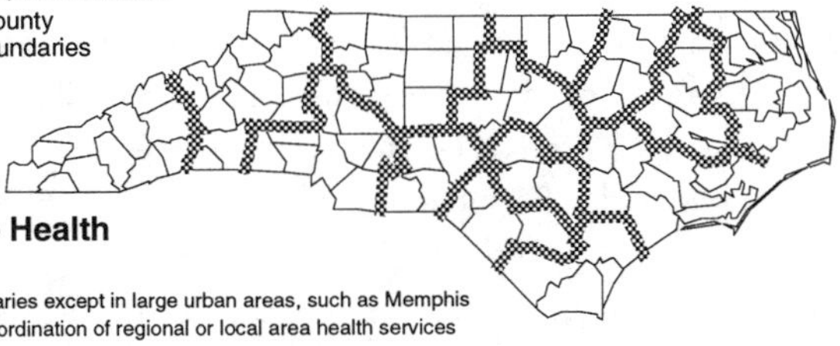

1966
Comprehensive Health Planning Areas
- Followed political boundaries except in large urban areas, such as Memphis
- Developed to support coordination of regional or local area health services

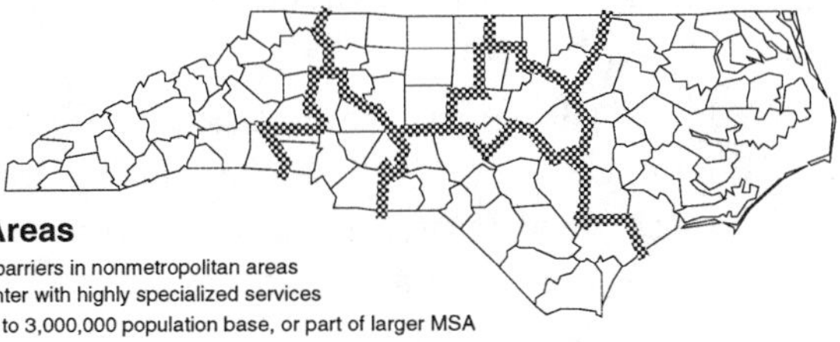

1974
Health Service Areas
- Considered geographic barriers in nonmetropolitan areas
- Included at least one center with highly specialized services
- Developed with 500,000 to 3,000,000 population base, or part of larger MSA

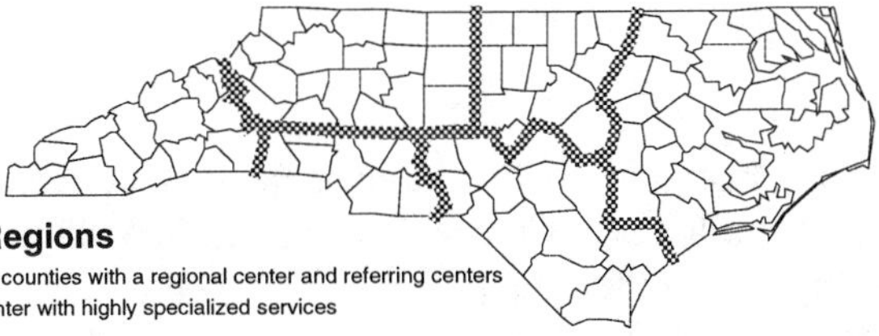

1977
Perinatal Care Regions
- Consisted of contiguous counties with a regional center and referring centers
- Included at least one center with highly specialized services

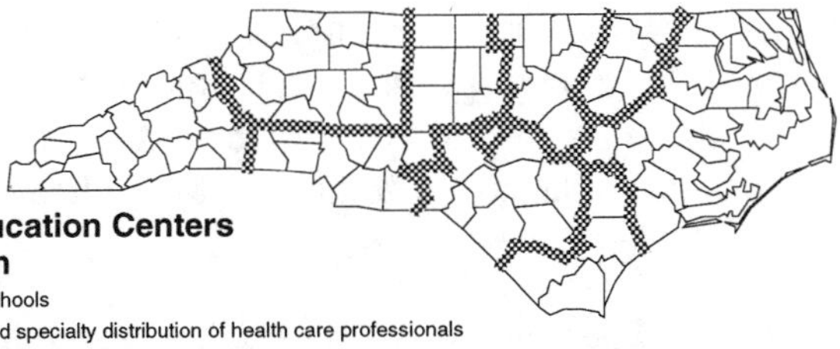

1977
Area Health Education Centers (AHEC) Program
- Located near medical schools
- Improved geographic and specialty distribution of health care professionals
- Improved accessibility to continuing education and to other health care professionals

Sources: Florin, 1980. In: *Conceptual and Methodological Issues in Medical Geography;*
NC Perinatal Care Regionalization Advisory Council, 1975. Regionalized Perinatal Health
Care Program of the NC Department of Human Resources, Division of Health Services;
and Odegaard, 1980. *Eleven Area Health Education Centers: The View from the Grass Roots.*

Figure 6-2   **Health Service Area Regionalization Plans Developed Under Block Grants**

services associated with comprehensive health planning and public health services (Figure 6-2). In the two decades after the Hill-Burton Act, most federal funds given to states had been in the form of categorical grants—that is, for a specific purpose. That approach was criticized as too rigid, denying the states flexibility to determine how best to use their funds. The Comprehensive Health Planning (CHP) and Public Health Services Amendments of 1966 (Public Laws 89-749) established Comprehensive Health Planning Agencies and provided for "block" grants to meet this criticism. To qualify, states had to provide an acceptable plan. Grants were authorized for developing regional, metropolitan area or other local plans.

Nearly all CHP areas were established along county lines, usually with groups of counties. They sometimes crossed state boundaries, usually to accommodate large urban areas such as St. Louis (combining areas of Missouri and Illinois), or Washington, DC (incorporating parts of Virginia and Maryland). Federal support for Comprehensive Health Planning was completely eliminated in 1986.

Health Service Areas (HSAs)

The National Health Planning and Resources Development Act of 1974 built on the Comprehensive Health Planning legislation by calling for regional planning areas. These were often congruent with the CHP areas and in some instances crossed state borders. Although federal funding of the Act ended in 1986, some states continue to have health planning and in many of those HSAs are still used for allocating resources using Certificate of Need (CON) laws or for proactive planning efforts. North Carolina is an example of the former, New York, the latter.

Area Health Education Centers (AHEC) Program

The Area Health Education Centers Program was established in 1971 to encourage the establishment or maintenance of training programs to alleviate health professional shortages. The AHECs that developed linked health care providers to central health sciences centers or functioned as community-based consortia of providers and training institutions. In the North Carolina AHEC, an early grantee, staff from the medical school visit regional AHEC hospitals for short terms to provide both training and health care. These hospitals are larger, often tertiary care centers located centrally in the regions. Medical or other health science students may spend longer periods of time at the AHEC hospitals. Funds are provided to these regional hospitals for general improvements and to develop regional medical education programs.

The AHEC programs which were created are strongly hierarchical, focused upon the university medical centers. Program boundaries follow county lines and, in almost all instances, state borders (Figure 6-2). A significant exception is the Washington, Alaska, Montana, Idaho (WAMI) AHEC and educational support network which includes the four states in one AHEC.

Perinatal Care Regions

Many states constructed Perinatal Care Regions in the 1970's and 1980's to reduce perinatal and maternal mortality and to improve the health prospects of perinatal survivors. The delivery system that evolved was strongly hierarchical, with more difficult cases routinely referred to higher order centers in a three-tiered system. North Carolina put in place its Perinatal Care Regions in 1977 (Figure 6-2).

The perinatal care regions created loosely mirror this intensely hierarchical system. Each region was established to advise the state about the planning, implementation, and success of the perinatal program in that region. It was recognized that regions were different from one another, with the result that programs should be fitted to the needs of the particular region.

The perinatal care system has focused intense effort and attracted close scrutiny because the issue of excess perinatal and infant mortality has been recognized as an issue of major national concern for several decades. The American Medical Association argued for a regionalized (rationalized) system to meet that need in the early 1970's (Meyer, 1980). Other studies encouraged a similar development, one that some states had already initiated.

Figure 6-3   **North Carolina Hospitals Classified by Level of Perinatal Service, 1989**

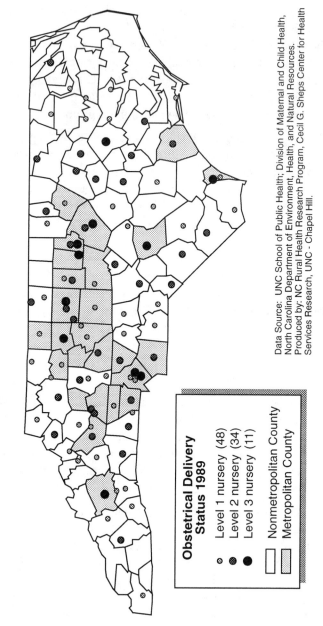

Obstetrical Delivery Status 1989

⊗ Level 1 nursery (48)
● Level 2 nursery (34)
● Level 3 nursery (11)

☐ Nonmetropolitan County
▨ Metropolitan County

Data Source: UNC School of Public Health; Division of Maternal and Child Health, North Carolina Department of Environment, Health, and Natural Resources.
Produced by: NC Rural Health Research Program, Cecil G. Sheps Center for Health Services Research, UNC - Chapel Hill.

The North Carolina Perinatal Care Program, like many others, identified a tiered system intended to insure minimum levels of acceptable accessibility (Figure 6-3). Level I centers, providing normal care for pregnant mothers and newborns, are to be within one hour of all patients. Level II centers, capable of meeting most high-risk pregnancy and newborn needs, are to be no more than two hours away. Level III centers, providing a complete program for all conditions, may be as much as three hours away. At least one Level III hospital was placed in each of the state's six perinatal regions, while at least a Level I program was to be in place in all facilities providing perinatal care. The program is also designed to encourage minimum cost with effective delivery of services. However, the 123 hospitals associated with the program were reduced to 93 between 1977 and 1990.

There are widespread indications that perinatal regionalization has reduced mortality (Tomich & Anderson, 1990; Mayfield et al., 1990). Obstetric and neonatal care regionalization has also encouraged innovative transportation efforts to achieve desired access to Level II and Level III centers. Helicopter transportation has been especially important. While expensive, such innovative efforts have proven effective in lowering mortality and are often cost-effective (Elliot et al., 1982).

On Constructing Regions

Which Regionalization Scheme to Use?

As mentioned earlier, there is no such thing as a "best" regionalization, and there is no one way to regionalize. Rather, any attempt at creating regions must first recognize and consider a series of critical issues.

Geographic Scale. Scale in the sense that geographers use the term simply refers to the size of the area under investigation. Scale, however, has a profound impact on the possibilities of regionalization. For example, health care regions cannot exist without an adequate resource base, so any regionalization system must consider available resources. That resource base is more often defined in terms of population size than geographic area. Thus, health care regions in densely populated areas may be much smaller with respect to geographic area than those in more sparsely populated areas. This is evident in the way counties in the western half of the United States are generally much larger than those in the East. A principle explanation for that difference is that the sparse population across much of the West often necessitated a larger county or state to assemble a population sufficiently large to support collective activities.

Scale can also affect the very questions one can ask, and, thus, the nature of useful data. Consider a regionalization of hospital use by patient residence. If the study includes all of a larger state, then it will likely be difficult to use data at any geographic unit other than the county. Given this scale, basic research and policy questions will focus upon inter-county patient flows to the hospitals. A program regionalizing a single county, or small group of counties, could by comparison use actual patient residence data at the street address level, creating a far more geographically detailed regionalization. Which is better? Again, neither one. The answer to that must depend on the research question—what you are trying to investigate.

As a related issue, data collected and regionalized at one level of geographic aggregation, or one scale of regionalization, should not be used to make observations about conditions at another geographic scale. Such comparisons should only be made among observations made at the same scale. To do otherwise is to commit what is called an ecological fallacy, that is, ascribing the general characteristics of a population to its individuals or ascribing invalid causes or associations based on aggregate data.

Spatial Contiguity. Should all of the territory within a region be geographically contiguous? There is no single answer to that question. Contiguity is often an advantage for planning purposes. It is usually easier to deal with a contiguous environment. Still, the world is often not organized in such a neat fashion. Physicians frequently have patients come from different geographic sectors of the community; this is the result of referral practices, ties of ethnicity or religion, residence, or any of a host of other possibilities. Programs aimed at economically impoverished portions of a community often discover that the poor do not all live in the same area. Sometimes contiguity should be ignored to create the most appropriate regionalization.

Political Borders as Regional Boundaries. As we noted in the discussion of the historical development of health care regionalization in the United States, regional boundaries often follow political—most often county or state—borders. There are two explanations for this common pattern. First, activity (for example, block grants or facilities planning) is often implemented within the context of such specified political units. Second, they are easy to use. Such borders are readily located, most individuals and agencies know in which political unit they are found, and many forms of data from the US Bureau of the Census and other agencies are made readily available based on these political units. Third, they are associated with tax collections and the subsequent distribution of government funds. This factor strongly influences structures and relationships.

There are disadvantages with the use of political borders for many kinds of regional boundaries, however. Most importantly, many kinds of human behavior ignore them. People select their health care units with little regard for such divisions; these can be called normative regions. This is also true for the distribution of health conditions, from poverty to the pattern of spread of an infectious disease. The problem of identifying correct location can be much greater if political boundaries are ignored, but sometimes the effort is necessary.

Many political units lack homogeneity; a county may contain a large city with its great social and economic diversity, as well as substantial rural areas that are quite different from the city. That lack of homogeneity presents both a boundary problem and a scale issue. Data for the entire county comprise an average, and will tend to mask the great variety of conditions found there. A regionalization that treats that county as a single unit has inherent problems.

Sometimes the investigator has no choice, but use of that regionalization scheme should be done with recognition of its limitations.

Changing Trends in Migration and Activity Spaces. Any regionalization should be viewed as temporary. People move, sometimes in large numbers. Neighborhoods age or change economically or ethnically. Rural areas become suburbs. Peoples' activity spaces, the territory they commonly use on an almost daily basis, change. Such change is a part of geography. Thus, regions created to define and meet the needs of that shifting population must also change. This holds for the clinic that defines its own patient origin area or the state creating a system to meet the broad needs of its population.

Relevance and Logic with Respect to Application. If we accept the statement that there is no such thing as the most correct regionalization—that the issue has meaning only within the context of the specific purpose of the regional scheme—then a responsibility of the regionalizer is to ask if the regionalization is relevant and logical. Am I using the right data? Am I using appropriate boundaries? Is the scale correct? In general, it is appropriate to use the simplest approach that meets those criteria.

Other Ways to Construct Regions

There are a variety of methods that can be used to construct regions. We will look at just a few of them here. Our focus is upon methods that demand little in the way of complex cartographic equipment and software, as well as limited sophistication in statistical techniques.

Theissen Polygons. A major problem with regional delimitation is boundary location. It is often rather easy to locate the core of a region, but its margins may be less clearly defined. Theissen polygons provide a method of at least roughly anticipating the boundaries of nodal regions with very little data. The use of this technique may be appropriate when considering the regions surrounding a number of nodal centers. The only data that are needed are the locations of the nodal centers themselves. A basic premise in the use of Thiessen polygons is that nodal region boundaries are found

Figure 6-4   **Level III Obstetrical Delivery Hospital Regions,1989**
(Constructed Using Thiessen Polygons)

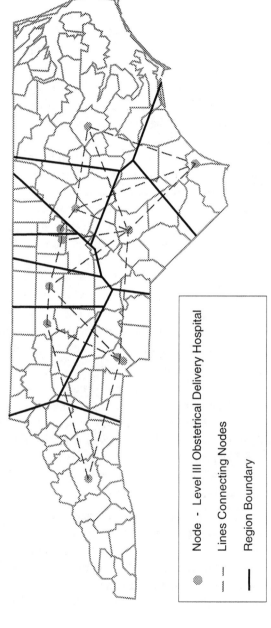

Node - Level III Obstetrical Delivery Hospital

Lines Connecting Nodes

Region Boundary

Data Sources: UNC School of Public Health; NC Division of Maternal and Child Health, NC Department of Environment, Health, and Natural Resources.
Produced by: NC Rural Health Research Program, Cecil G. Sheps Center for Health Services Research, UNC - Chapel Hill.

midway between nodal centers. Such a system allocates areas to the nearest node, without regard to any interfering barriers or preferences.

Consider the distribution of Level III obstetrical hospitals discussed earlier and shown in Figure 6-3. The 11 hospitals are located in ten communities. Polygon construction begins with the construction of lines connecting each adjacent or nearby pair. This demands some decision making. Charlotte and Asheville in the west are clearly adjacent in that there is no other Level III community between them. But, what about Charlotte and Raleigh? A line between them passes through no other Level III node, but there are nearby nodes to the north and south. A simple solution to the problem is to try both—a regionalization assuming that connection and one that does not. Once the join lines are drawn, construct perpendicular lines bisecting each join line at its midpoint. Extend these perpendiculars until they meet another perpendicular line. These perpendiculars form the Theissen polygon regional boundaries and, thus, map the regional pattern (Figure 6-4). It is often necessary to reconstruct the boundary system several times to construct an acceptable regionalization. Some joins may just have been inappropriate because of topographical barriers, cultural or linguistic patterns, or a misreading of the equivalence of the nodes.

To restate, the value of a regionalization based on Theissen polygons derives from the minimal data required and the relative ease of construction. There are no utilization data required for its construction. Because these regions are based solely on existing locations of health care facilities, some of which may be obsolete or inappropriately used, additional information would have to be collected to "prove" their appropriateness. Still, the basic assumption—that use is assigned to the nearest node—has considerable validity.

Flow Maps. Flow maps in health care commonly present the pattern of movement of patients from the place of origin, usually their residence, to a care center. As such, they define patterns of nodal activity. As mentioned earlier, such maps are often used to define the service region for a single center. They can also be used to regionalize a larger area.

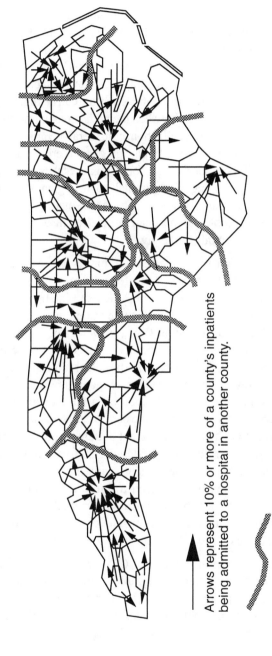

Figure 6-5 **North Carolina Acute Care Hospital Patient Origins, 1989**

Arrows represent 10% or more of a county's inpatients being admitted to a hospital in another county.

The shaded lines represent visual isoclines separating apparent service areas.

Data Source: North Carolina Division of Facility Services, Hospital Patient Origin Book, 1990.
Produced by: NC Rural Health Research Program, Cecil G. Sheps Center for Health Services Research, UNC - Chapel Hill.

The accompanying map of inter-county hospital patient flows in North Carolina presents the pattern of movement of individuals for all inpatient admissions at short-term, acute care hospitals in 1989 (Figure 6-5). (A similar flow map is Figure 4-2 in Chapter 4.) Lines or vectors identify the most significant inter-county flows as a percentage of all such hospitalizations from each county. The state can be regionalized by simply drawing boundaries between the nodal concentrations. As with a Theissen polygon regionalization, considerable variation in the pattern of regions can be achieved by changing the criteria for assigning centers or nodes. This regionalization, for example, centers on the more dominant hospitals, assigning lesser hospitals to the region of that more dominant central hospital. However, these movement patterns may reflect accessibility problems where patients with no insurance may be forced to travel to hospitals farther away.

Overlay Maps. We mentioned earlier that regions can be either single-featured or multifeatured. Multifeatured regions can present a challenging construction. How does one examine these various features? How are they interrelated? Such issues can be addressed with various statistical techniques or a powerful new computer-based cartographic approach commonly called Geographic Information Systems (GIS), but they can also be at least considered using simpler cartographic techniques. Overlay mapping is an example. Suppose that a nodal region is defined by a number of different activities, each with its own distinctive pattern. One instance of this might be a clinic with distinctly different patient origin patterns for each of the various services it provides. Each use pattern can be mapped on a separate transparent sheet, using the same base map. The entire set can then be overlayed to build a "picture" of the clinic's service region, identifying the area for which the clinic is a dominant center for a majority of its provided services and the area for which only one or a few of its services are important.

Geographic Information Systems (GIS). Geographic information systems essentially join cartography, multivariate statistical analysis, and the computer to create the opportunity for effective analysis of a complex variety of geographic data. The statistical analysis component of a GIS allows the investigator to classify (regionalize) and portray data in innovative ways. Many GIS software programs are available for both personal computers and larger machines. GIS, already important, promises to become a central method in geography-based planning over the next few years.

The integration of health services research with GIS technologies offers promise in examining complex issues through a process that includes input, storage and retrieval, manipulation and analysis, and output (maps, charts, and reports) of geographic data (Twigg, 1990). Cowen (1990) further refines the definition of GIS, seeing it as "a decision support system involving the integration of spatially referenced data in a problem solving environment." The use of GIS facilitates a quantitative approach (Verhasselt, 1993) and has the potential to further knowledge in the health sciences in "quantum jumps" (Matthews, 1990). See the Point of Departure at the end of this chapter for a more in-depth discussion of GIS.

Health Service Areas from Cluster Analysis. Diane Makuc and others have recently developed a health care service regionalization of the entire United States using 1988 Medicare patient origin data on short-term hospital stays (Makuc et al., 1991). The county is the minimum unit largely because use of any smaller unit created too many locations for geographic analysis at the national level. ZIP code information or Census tract data might have allowed a more geographically detailed effort if they had focused their work on a smaller area. A hierarchical cluster analysis approach was used to collapse the over 3,000 US counties into a smaller number of regions. Hierarchical clustering joins units (counties in this case) in an iterative process based on their similarities. That is, the two most similar units in terms of the data used are joined, then the next two most similar, until eventually the entire set of units is joined into a single group. A geographic contiguity constraint can be included in the analysis. The investigation can use any of a number of different approaches to stop the process at any desired level of regionalization. Makuc chose to develop about 800 regions.

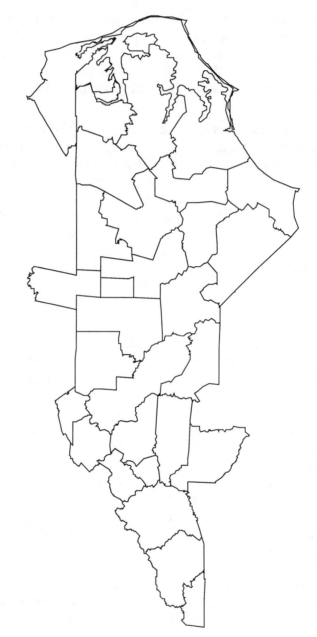

Figure 6-6   **Health Service Areas in North Carolina**

Data Source: National Center for Health Statistics, Vital and Health Statistics, Health Service Areas for the United States 1991, Series 2, No. 112.

The Makuc et al. regionalization follows county boundaries but ignores state boundaries (Figure 6-6). It creates a loosely nodal pattern in that many of the regions focus around significant urban centers. Makuc chose her level of regionalization based on a mathematical algorithm. She could have used alternative numbers to solve the clustering problem; she settled on 800 because it reduced the variance in her summary measure. Different solutions could be more or less helpful in different parts of the country based on variance in existing conditions or levels.

Some Summary Comments

This chapter has introduced notions of regions and regionalization, and suggested several approaches to region building. Regionalization has been as much a philosophical point of view in health care delivery as it has been a practical guide to the organization of services. Regional systems have appeared as a result of market forces as often as they have derived from planned regional structures or programs. The extension of the vertical scale of complexity in health care, which is a result of technology building, is causing more and more spatial concentration of services. This concentration is stimulating the growth of regional arrangements as high technology becomes clustered into central places and services of diminishing complexity distribute themselves around those central places.

Regionalization will become much more important in the financial structure of health systems as continuous pressure for reform identifies bounded areas where limited competition is allowed. This pressure for the creation of regions or areas may draw on the methods described here, but more likely will react to political geography as much as to the recognition that efficiency does not necessarily respect boundaries.

▷P O I N T
▷OF DEPARTURE

Rural Places and Regionalization
John Florin

Person County lies along the northern border of North Carolina in the rolling Piedmont country of the central part of the state. The county's population is just over 30,000, with fewer than 10,000 in the county seat of Roxboro. The county is relatively poor, as are most predominantly rural sections of the state. Most jobs are in agriculture (the county lies in the famous Bright Leaf tobacco belt), in one of the many small manufacturing firms found mostly in Roxboro, or in service industries. Many workers commute 35 miles south to jobs in the booming cities of the central Piedmont or in "the Park," the Research Triangle Park between Raleigh and Durham. Over 15 percent of the county's residents do not have health insurance, compared with 12.4 percent for the entire state.

The county's single hospital, Person County Memorial Hospital, is located in Roxboro, and by 1990 it was in trouble. It operated 54 beds in 1989, and is run by a non-profit association as are a majority of North Carolina's rural hospitals. As recently as 1980, the average bed occupancy rate for the hospital had been 77.9 percent; in 1989, it had fallen to 36.4 percent—far below the state-set target of 75 percent for hospitals of its size. Almost 60 percent of all 1989 discharges were for patients aged 65 or above. In 1980, 19 physicians were affiliated with the hospital; by 1989, that number had fallen to ten. The hospital's lone OB/GYN in 1980 was gone by 1989. Perhaps most telling, the share of all NC hospital discharges for Person County residents from Person County Memorial had fallen from over 46 to 27.2 percent. The Hospital was not seen as the preferred place for care by many residents of the county and the loss of providers reduced admissions because patients went elsewhere for diagnosis. One result was that, in 1989, the hospital suffered an operating loss of over $900,000 (Lambrew & Betts, 1991; Harris, 1991).

What was happening at Person County Memorial? First, many of the changes were not unique to that hospital. Three of the 78 rural hospitals in North Carolina in 1980 had closed by 1990, and the expectation was that a number of others would follow that course in the 1990's. These closures in North Carolina were reflected nationally. Over 500 rural hospitals shut their doors in the 1980's. The map in Figure 6-7 locates these closed facilities. Average hospital use nationally declined by over 11 percent during the 1980's. In North Carolina and nationally, rural hospitals suffered a decline in occupancy rates that was more than twice that average. This was partly due to a national recession, but more the result of changing federal and insurance company policies—most notably the Prospective Payment System introduced by Medicare that created financial incentives for the early discharge of patients relative to recommended lengths of stay for specified disease groups called Diagnosis-Related Groups (DRGs).

The mix of users at a typical rural hospital also changed during the decade. Rural hospitals are increasingly used by older, poorer patients as the demographic structure in most rural communities ages. The young and more affluent rural residents will tend to travel some distance to usually larger, urban hospitals to obtain needed care, just as they journey to those same cities for a variety of shopping and employment activities. Both the rural hospital and the traditional small town main street business have suffered as a consequence.

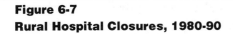

Figure 6-7
Rural Hospital Closures, 1980-90

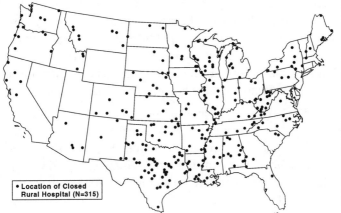

• Location of Closed
Rural Hospital (N=315)

Data Source: Hospital Closure File 1980-89, Health Database
Services, American Hospital Association. Hospital Closure 1990,
Office of Inspector General, DHHS.

Others have suggested that another cause of the declining use of rural hospitals such as Person County Memorial is the growing significance of regionalization—the careful and planned allocation of new health care resources. Regionalization in this case is defined as "...a process which optimizes access to technology. Regionalization is based on a tiered structure of facilities linked by referral patterns..." (Mayfield et al., 1990). In this case the centripetal forces of regionalization dominated. Moreover, regionalization has been fostered by the rapid growth of high-cost technology and the desire to see it diffuse rationally according to need. In North Carolina, the acquisition of high-level technology (e.g., Magnetic Resonance Image [MRI] machines) is controlled through a Certificate of Need (CON) system which requires justification for the addition of new capital equipment and additional capacity in excess of fixed amounts. This mandated health care regionalization emphasized larger (and often more urban) hospitals in the investment of limited health care resources. Smaller (and often more rural) hospitals were limited in their ability to add new technology or replace capital, with the result that those hospitals quickly became outdated, appearing less desirable to the "shopping" public and to physicians making referrals. The hospitals were also less likely to have management trained to cope with these changes and fewer physicians who felt these hospitals could meet their needs.

Person County is an example of a health care facility that could function in a regionalized system, but the prevailing trend is toward centralization. Regional structures have to function in both directions with referrals flowing to the center and non-referral patients remaining with nearby "regional" caregivers.

▷ P O I N T
▷ OF DEPARTURE

Geographic Information Systems (GIS)

Don Albert

GIS is an acronym for Geographic Information System, which, in simple terms, combines geography with other data. Geographic Information System (GIS) is a generic name for other descriptive terms such as Land Information System (LIS), Land and Resource Information System (LRIS), Urban Information System (URIS), Environmental Information System (ERIS), Cadastral Information System (CAIS), and Geographic Information Processing (GIP) (Taylor, 1991).

While there is no universally accepted definition of GIS (Martin, 1991; Taylor, 1991), the following generally reflects the range of common usage in both academic and professional circles. Geographic Information Systems are manual or computer databases that store and manipulate geographic referenced data (Aronoff, 1989), that is, data that are linked to geographic descriptors like latitude and longitude or a boundary system. A GIS can also be defined in terms of its five basic subcomponents: 1) data input and editing, 2) data management, 3) data query and retrieval, 4) data analysis/modeling/synthesis, and 5) data display and output (Parr, 1991). The International City Management Association (1991) defines GIS as a "computer system of hardware and software that integrates graphics with databases and allows for display, analysis, and modeling," while the Federal Interagency Coordinating Committee's definition emphasizes the usefulness of such geographic information in "solving complex planning and management problems" (Antenucci et al., 1991). Star and Estes (1990) coined the term the "four M's" in their definition of GIS, referring to its measurement, mapping, monitoring, and modeling capabilities.

Cowen (1990) asserts that defining the standard components of GIS as: input, storage and retrieval, manipulation, and output is overly general and thus inadequate. He states that it is the capacity to *integrate* geographic information that constitutes a GIS, specifically through the *polygon overlay* process which he sees as its defining aspect. This integrative process is more inclusive than merely combining separate layers of information (e.g., roads, school locations, railroad routes) to form a composite map, and rather produces new information through the integration of multiple layers of spatial and demographic data. The polygon overlay process consists of: 1) overlaying two or more maps comprised of polygons, which usually represent boundaries or physical features of a land area (layer #1 and layer #2 in Figure 6-8), 2) determining the intersection of these polygons, and 3) using this intersection to form resultant polygons (intersection of layers 1 and 2 in Figure 6-8). The potential for integrating spatial data in such a manner sets GIS apart from other methods of computer mapping.

Cowen's rationale for GIS as polygon integration draws on the Geographical Matrix concept developed by Brian Berry in the 1960's (1964). This matrix conceptualizes the discipline in terms of systematic (e.g., climatology, geomorphology, political, economic) and regional geography (Figure 6-9). The rows of the matrix are societal and physical characteristics and the columns are places. In the geographical matrix shown in Figure 6-9, the examination of one characteristic (or row), e.g., population, for various places (or columns), here, for example, Asheville, Canton, Robbinsville, Sylva, and Waynesville, North Carolina, comprises a systematic geographical approach. Conversely, the examination of societal/physical characteristics (e.g., population, hospitals, physician offices, street networks, and zoning) looking down

Figure 6-8
Integration of Spatial Data with Polygon Overlay Process

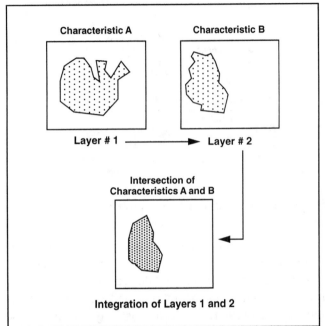

Characteristic A   Characteristic B

Layer # 1 ——————→ Layer # 2

Intersection of
Characteristics A and B

Integration of Layers 1 and 2

one column (e.g., Asheville, North Carolina) is a regional geographical approach. The latter approach underscores the theoretical basis for Cowen's definition of GIS. Essentially each row/column intersection can be thought of as a map consisting of polygons defining regions. Two or more row/column intersections within the same column can be integrated through the polygon overlay process to create resultant regions (as shown in Figure 6-9), which then convey information about several variables regarding the resultant area or activity space. This capability suggests the great potential for the use of GIS in providing useful and timely information for policy makers. Cowen states that a "GIS is ... a decision support system involving the integration

Figure 6-9
Geographical Matrix

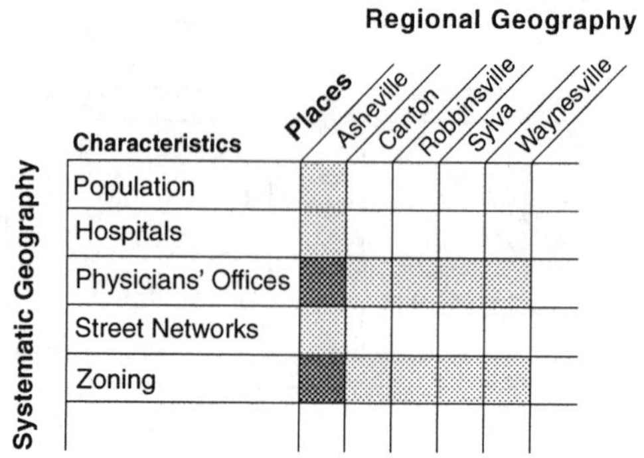

of spatially referenced data in a problem solving environment" (Cowen, 1990).

The integration of the geography of health, including health care delivery and disease ecology, with GIS technologies offers enormous potential. GIS can provide the basis for a "quantum jump" in our ability to understand the connections between health status and geography because it is so powerful and flexible (Matthews, 1990). To date, the literature on health research and GIS remains rather scarce, but is growing rapidly. Recent contributions to the literature have tended to focus on both possible (theoretical) and actual (practical) uses of GIS to investigate the spatial components of health care research.

The following are examples of applications reported recently (see Table 6-1): Lam (1986) suggests using a GIS to analyze geographical patterns of cancer mortality in the almost 2,400 counties of China. The necessary data for this would include age- and sex-specific rates of cancer along with environmental and socioeconomic variables; the large amount of data required for this sort of epidemiologic analysis would mandate the use of a GIS (Matthews, 1990). Wartenberg

Table 6-1
Applications of Geographic Information
Systems to Health Research

Author(s)	Question	Geography	Variables
Lam (1986)	analyze cancer mortality	identify spatial patterns	cancer rates socioeconomic (age, race, sex) environmental (air and water pollution)
Guthe (1992)	prediction of high blood lead levels among children	identification of high-risk census tracks	blood screening records local sources of industrial and hazardous wastes traffic volume
Stallones et al. (1992)	reproductive outcomes surveillance	proximity to hazardous waste sites	low birth weight hazardous waste sites
Wartenberg (1992)	development of lead-screening program	identification of high-risk neighborhoods	population density SES water supply age of housing industrial sources
Zwarenstein et al. (1991)	measuring accessibility	defining hospital catchment areas	persons/bed ratios

P
O
I
N
T

O
F

D
E
P
A
R
T
U
R
E

(1992) has envisioned the development of a lead screening program using a GIS that identifies high-incidence neighborhoods based on risk factors such as population density (high), socio-economic status (low), water supply (lead solder), age of housing (old) and proximity to local industrial sources of lead. Stallones et al. (1992) propose using GIS in surveillance of reproductive outcomes (e.g., low birth weight) around hazardous waste sites. Guthe et al. (1992) ran a pilot project using a GIS to compare the expected versus actual spatial pattern of the occurrence of high blood lead levels among children in Newark, East Orange, and Irving, New Jersey. The findings exposed some differences in the expected versus actual spatial pattern, suggesting that additional parameters are needed for more accurate prediction of high-risk census tracts. Zwarenstein et al. (1991) delimited hypothetical hospital catchment districts for Natal/KwaZulu in South Africa with Thiessen polygons using a GIS. The results showed that the removal of race restrictions on hospital admissions in 1985 did not improve the person/bed ratio for blacks.

These uses of GIS in a health context point to its ability to bring together complex information describing exposure, facilities/provider use, and disease information to assist policy makers in their decisions. The spread of GIS into health services research has been rapid in the sense that it has been used so quickly after becoming generally available. Its complete utility is yet to be realized, however, because data access is so problematic in the health care system. In addition, the large data files that are usually required necessitate access to a computer with a great deal of both storage space and processing capability. As data gathering improves and regional and national systems are implemented, GIS can approach its potential in health care.

Chapter 7

Methods for Defining Medical Service Areas

Point of Departure:
Hospital Closure and Access to Hospital Services

Background

The use of ecologic analysis is of increasing interest to a growing number of researchers because, in many cases, the use of group or population data may be the only practical method to answer important questions regarding certain types of policy decisions. Individual-level data are expensive to obtain and, for many questions that relate to past events, essentially impossible to capture. Research examining group- or population-level data will likely increase in coming years because variations in access to care and cost, effectiveness, or quality of care can be discovered by examining differences between defined populations. One common way to identify population groups of interest in ecologic analysis is by examining differences between populations living in specific medical service areas.

Medical service areas must be carefully defined in order to be useful for analysis. Each of the methods currently used to define medical service areas is based on a different set of assumptions regarding the utilization of care, and each is appropriate to answer only certain types of research questions. Because no method will provide us with the perfect set of boundaries for a population of interest, the advantages and disadvantages of each method must be considered for each study on an individual basis.

Wright and Marlor (1990) have identified over two dozen methods of medical service area definition in the literature. Of these, three are most commonly applied in health services research: geographical methods, geopolitical methods, and patient origin methods (Garnick et al., 1987). Most published studies using medical service areas examine hospital–patient relationships. Wright and Marlor (1990) address the need for correspondence between the purpose of the analysis and the conceptual framework of a particular technique.

A number of researchers have discussed different market area definition methodologies and their applications. Stano (1993) points out that, to date, most inter-area studies of utilization use an inappropriately broad market area definition and range of diagnoses. Garnick et al. (1987) argue that all methods of medical service area definition need to be refined and that different methodologies are appropriate to different situations.

Only recently have the consequences of different methodologies on size and composition of defined market areas been closely examined. Garnick et al. (1987) point out that patient origin methods typically yield medical service areas that contain fewer competitive providers than those defined using geopolitical and geographic methods. Goody (1993b) compared geopolitically-defined (in this case county-based) medical service areas to patient origin-defined medical service areas and found that county-based medical service areas are four times too large (i.e., they include areas from which the study hospital does not draw patients). Goody did, however, find that socioeconomic and demographic characteristics are very similar in patient origin and geopolitical medical service areas. This limited research reveals some of the problems associated with different market area definition methods and illustrates that we need to understand them better before we can effectively use ecologic analysis.

This chapter describes the three major methods of service area definition: 1) the geographic distance method, which uses measurements of fixed distance from patient residence or physician office to a facility; 2) the geopolitical method, which uses preexisting geopolitical boundaries; and 3) the patient origin method, which is based on the distribution of patients using a facility. Apart from developing methods, research employing medical service areas can be classified into three categories: planning/predictive, descriptive, and evaluative. We examine possible combinations of medical service area definition methods with research purposes and discuss the appropriate matching of method to application. A number of criteria provide guidance in the selection of appropriate methods of service area definition for different kinds of research. We describe these criteria and discuss their applicability to each medical service area definition method.

Medical Service Areas Defined by
Geographic Distance

The geographic distance method of medical service area definition includes in a service area the population that lives or works within a specified distance of a source of care. An example of a geographic distance medical service area is the area described by a fifty-mile radius around a study hospital (Figure 7-1). This method is based on the concept that, for a relatively homogeneous population, the utilization of a hospital's services declines as the real or perceived "cost" of accessing the services increases (Morrill & Earickson, 1968); from a geography perspective, this follows central place theory and the concept of distance decay.

Studies of the relationship between travel distance and medical service utilization were conducted as early as the 1930's. However,

Figure 7-1
Geographic Distance Method of Medical Service
Area Definition

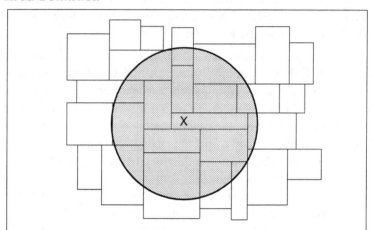

Counties Surrounding an Index Hospital. The circle delineates a
fifty-mile radius from the index hospital. Each of the boxes represents
a county.

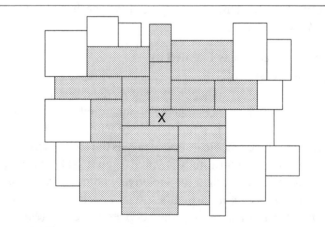

Geographically Defined Medical Service Area (MSA). Shaded
boxes represent counties that fell within a fifty-mile radius; shaded
boxes are within MSA. Unshaded boxes represent counties that
did not fall within a fifty-mile radius; unshaded boxes are not within
the MSA. When less than ten percent of a county fell within the
fifty-mile radius, the county was not included in the MSA.

the enactment of the Hospital Survey and Construction (Hill-Burton) Act of 1946 accelerated the pace of such studies by holding out the first real promise that they would be answered with policy initiatives for locating facilities in underserved areas. In 1954, Ciocco and Altman were the first to develop a quantitative index of medical service areas that included a measure of the distances that patients traveled for care (Shannon et al., 1969). In a joint report released in 1961, the American Hospital Association and the Public Health Service stated that travel time and transportation consider-ations should be used in health facility planning (Shannon et al., 1969). Lubin, Drosness and Wylie (1965) also demonstrated the value of travel distance information to health planning with the development of their Highway Network Minimum Path Selection approach to facility location decisions (Shannon et al., 1969).

More recently, the geographic distance method of medical service area definition has been employed not only to look at resource allocation and the need for hospital construction, but also to study competition for clients among neighboring hospitals, variation in distances that patients travel for different kinds of hospital services, and patterns of physician affiliations with hospi-tals. Luft and Maerki (1984-85) described geographic service areas using two different estimates of the distance that physicians are willing to travel to supervise patient care. This study defined "neighborhoods," or areas where competition could occur, with both 5- and 15-mile radii to investigate the potential for competition among hospitals for physician affiliation.

Phibbs and Robinson (1993) compared ZIP code-based service areas and a variable radius measure of California hospital service areas to determine if the easier-to-construct radius measure could be used to identify hospital markets nationally. The project calculated the distance between the most distant ZIP code centroids that included 75 and 90 percent of each hospital's discharges and the location of the hospital. Using a regression technique, the project identified characteristics of the hospitals that could predict the radius. Com-parisons of the predicted service areas and the actual (ZIP code-based patient flow) areas produced reasonable correlations and led Phibbs and Robinson to conclude that the variable radius approach was a feasible and cost-effective way to construct hospital market areas until more sophisticated patient flow systems could be put into place.

Medical service areas defined by geographic distance have been used successfully in descriptive and planning-oriented research. This method is relatively simple and inexpensive to use. It also has the advantage of defining a unique market area for each facility studied. However, there are a number of drawbacks associated with the geographic distance method of medical service area definition. Medical service areas defined by fixed distances from a facility do not account for physical barriers to access such as rivers, lakes, mountains, or lack of highways or public transportation. On a more subtle note, although geographic distance can be a good proxy for travel time to a facility, this may differ from perceived travel time, which can be affected by lack of familiarity with the route to a hospital or other phenomena related to human effort, and can affect a person's decision to use services (Shannon et al., 1969).

Researchers using the geographic distance approach to medical service area definition should also be aware of the fact that different geographic distances are appropriate for different medical services. The distances that patients are willing to travel, or over which physicians will refer, vary depending upon whether the services in question are convenience goods (e.g., routine general care), shopping goods (e.g., obstetrical deliveries), or specialty goods (e.g., coronary artery bypass operations). The concept of distance decay formally addresses this phenomenon for various medical care services (Meade, Florin & Gesler, 1988). If physician referral patterns are not consistent with distance criteria, then the use of geographic distance service area definition may not be appropriate for studies of referrals in conjunction with patient travel.

A final consideration in the use of geographic distance to define medical service areas is the differences between rural and urban service areas. Independent service areas, or near-monopoly situations, are likely to be found only in rural areas, where there are few or no alternative facilities within a reasonable distance. Medical service areas defined in urban areas, on the other hand, are likely to contain multiple hospitals and therefore will usually reflect a high level of competition among hospitals. Therefore, geographic distance methods are usually more appropriate for defining medical service areas in rural areas.

Medical Service Areas Defined by Geopolitical Boundaries

Geopolitical medical service areas are defined by the boundaries of official governmental or regulatory units, such as counties, planning regions, states or nations, or aggregations of these. This definition is perhaps the oldest and most common way to identify unique populations of interest in order to examine differences in utilization or outcomes that may be related to provider characteristics. The concept underlying the use of this medical service area definition is that of public authority and accountability for monitoring and/or assuring population health.

The selection of a specific geopolitical unit to define population groups must be guided by the geographic area for which a decision maker, or group, has responsibility and fiscal authority. Thus, each medical service area should be no larger than the area for which decisions on resources allocations are made, and, if possible, subdivided to one level lower than the geographic area of responsibility (e.g., townships as part of counties). This smaller unit definition allows the researcher to examine variations in the measures of interest both within and among areas which are affected by decisions. This means that a medical service area should be defined at, or below, the level of a county if regulatory or fiscal responsibility is located at the county level.

In personal health services markets have most often been described in terms of the most common political subdivision for which data are easily available, the county (see Figure 7-2). Diane Makuc et al. (1985) used aggregations of counties to define service areas for hospital care. She found that this type of area had few

Figure 7-2

Geopolitical Boundary Method of Medical Service Area Definition

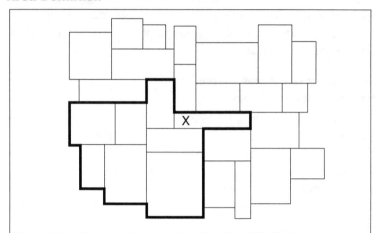

Townships Surrounding an Index Hospital. The X denotes the index hospital; each of the boxes represents a township. The boxes within the darker outline represent the townships comprising researcher's county of interest.

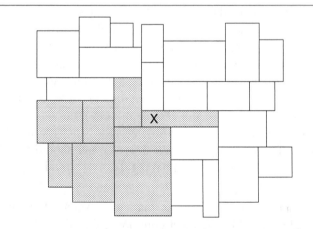

Geopolitically Defined Medical Service Area (MSA). Shaded boxes represent townships comprising researcher's county of interest; shaded boxes are within MSA. Unshaded boxes represent townships contained in other counties; unshaded boxes are not within the MSA.

patients seeking care outside the medical service area of origin, yet was able to capture variations in use rates. Dear (1977) used subsections of Lancaster County, Pennsylvania, to examine the relationship between the distance to mental health services and service use. His measures included four distance dimensions: physical distance, social distance, relative location, and catchment area specification.

Medical service area definition by geopolitical area has been used successfully in research that most often examines access, health outcomes, program effects, competition and a variety of issues that relate a public program or institution to a population. The focus on public programs is due to the general restriction of those to the borders of a political unit. The method is simple and relatively easy to use. Its strengths lie in the fact that many social, health, and economic measures are reported for geopolitical areas. This fact enables researchers to control for these factors when testing hypotheses. However, in many cases, private providers contribute significantly to the overall system of health care provision. These providers respond to policy and fiscal initiatives at variable rates and often have referral areas that do not correspond to geopolitical units. In such cases the use of geopolitical areas for defining medical service areas may not adequately capture the variations of interest.

Methodologically, relying on political geographies causes problems because these areas are fixed and of unequal sizes. Their rates have uneven variance, and this causes problems in comparison and complex analyses. In such cases, even relatively large areas may hold too small a population for a researcher to be able to identify significant differences in rates. This issue is demonstrated well in the attempt of Holahan and colleagues (1990) to measure variations in the level of physician services used by Medicare beneficiaries. These authors defined medical service areas for US states in terms of populations living in major metropolitan areas and those living in the rest of a state. Because they used a data set consisting of only a five percent sample of beneficiaries, they had inadequate power to measure differences in the use of several types of services for rural medical service areas. Researchers should carefully consider the influence of random variation in the rates of small population groups on study power when deciding to use a geopolitical medical service area definition.

Medical Service Areas Defined by the Patient Origin Method

Unlike geographic and geopolitical methods, the patient origin method represents actual utilization patterns (Figure 7-3). It also accounts for barriers to care and the structure of existing referral patterns. The patient origin method is also advantageous because it has the capability to calculate markets for subgroups of the population, e.g., Medicare patients (Garnick et al., 1987). However, it requires substantially larger amounts of data and more complex data manipulation and, therefore, has not been used in the literature as frequently as geographic and geopolitical methods. Nevertheless, most medium- to large-size facilities maintain in-house case mix systems that are used for planning purposes. Also 37 states have legislative mandates to maintain hospital-level databases that would facilitate this type of analysis. Lastly, Medicaid and HCFA Medicare databases can be used to construct medical service areas for select population subgroups.

The patient origin method looks at the care-seeking behavior of residents of small geographic areas (e.g., ZIP code areas). Each small area is assigned to a market area based on the behavior of its residents. "The ideal unit of analysis would have a population homogenous in all dimensions not explicitly figuring in the analysis. It would be small enough so that the medical care resources constitute a system in the sense that the population encounters a uniform set of arrangements for its care. Finally, service area boundaries would be impervious; the population would receive all of its medical care within the confines of the service area" (Wilson & Tedeschi, 1984). Unfortunately, such an ideal situation occurs rarely, if ever.

Figure 7-3
Patient Origin Method of Medical Service Area Definition

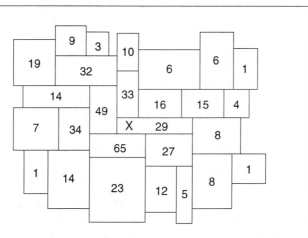

Zip Code Areas Surrounding an Index Hospital. Each box represents a ZIP code area with admissions to hospital X. The number in each box represents the total number of visits to hospital X originating from each ZIP code. There are 451 total admissions to hospital X.

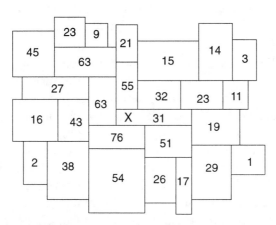

Number of Hospital Admissions To Any Hospital Originating From Each ZIP Code Area. The number in each box represents the total number of hospital visits to any hospital originating from each ZIP code. Any ZIP code sending a total of fewer than four admissions to any hospital is excluded from the MSA.

Because the ideal conditions are seldom met, researchers are forced to set criteria to determine whether a particular ZIP code should be included in or excluded from a medical service area. Measures of market share are typically the basis of these criteria. Griffith (1972) defines the institution–population relationship using two measures of market share: *relevance* and *commitment*. His index of relevance measures the proportion of total admissions by residents of an area to a particular hospital. The relevance index (RI) measures market share from the population perspective and is computed as:

$$RI = \frac{\text{number of admissions to hospital x from area y}}{\text{total admissions to any hospital from area y}}$$

Griffith's index of commitment measures the proportion of a hospital's admissions that are from a given area. Thus, the commitment index (CI) measures the importance of a defined geographic area as a patient source from the hospital's perspective and is computed as:

$$CI = \frac{\text{number of admissions to hospital x from area y}}{\text{total admissions to hospital x}}$$

Griffith's relevance and commitment indices are commonly used as the basis for inclusion criteria. For instance, in a medical service area defined from the population perspective (relevance), a ZIP code might be included in a medical service area if fifty percent of its admissions were to the hospital of interest. Another ZIP code might be excluded if only ten percent of its admissions were to the hospital of interest (see Figure 7-4). In a medical service area defined from the hospital perspective (commitment), a ZIP code might be included if ten percent of the hospital's total admissions were of residents of that ZIP code, but another ZIP code might be excluded if only one percent of the hospital's admissions were of residents of that ZIP code (see Figure 7-5). The two approaches can yield substantially different service areas.

Figure 7-4
Patient Origin Method of Medical Service Area
Definition: Relevance

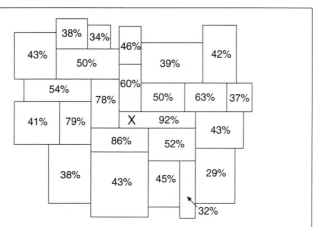

Percent of All Hospital Admissions in Each ZIP Code Area to Hospital of Interest. Proportion of admissions to hospital of interest drawn from each ZIP code area.

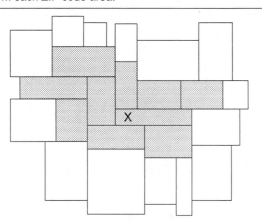

Patient Origin MSA Defined Using Relevance Index. Shaded boxes represent ZIP code areas where the index hospital has greater than or equal to 50% of market share; these areas fall within the medical service area (MSA). Unshaded boxes represent ZIP code areas where the index hospital has less than 50% of market share; these areas do not fall within the MSA.

Figure 7-5
Patient Origin Method of Medical Service Area
Definition: Commitment

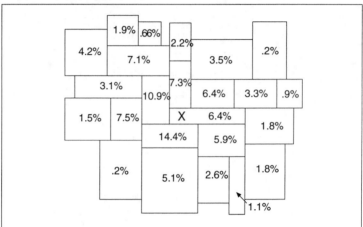

**Percent of Hospital of Interest's Total Admissions Originating in
Each ZIP Code Area.** Proportion of hospital of interest's patients
being drawn from each ZIP code area.
Note: Numbers may not total 100% due to rounding.

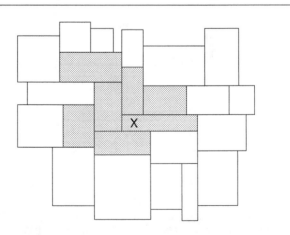

Patient Origin MSA Defined Using Commitment Index. ZIP code
areas are ranked by CI in descending order. ZIP code areas are
placed in the MSA in rank order until the MSA contains 60 percent of
all admissions to hospital X.

Zwanziger and Melnick (1988) defined service-specific market areas for individual hospitals using a measure of commitment. First, they identified all the ZIP code areas contributing at least three percent of a hospital's total discharges from that service category. Then, to ensure that diffuse market areas were not unduly truncated, they confirmed that the market area contained the ZIP codes that supplied the hospital with the largest number of discharges and that, together, made up at least forty percent of its discharges for that service.

Goody (1993a) used both a geopolitical boundary (the county) and two alternative boundaries (ZIP code-based commitment measures at 60 and 75 percent) to build service areas for 2,764 rural hospitals in a study of the correlates of closure. In general, the ZIP code-based service areas were much smaller than the county-based service areas, and there were important differences in total population and population density between the two groups. There was high correlation, however, among variables that described the race, age, income, unemployment, and migration patterns of the populations for the three types of market area. Goody's study illustrates the potential impact of service area definition methodology on size and sociodemographic makeup of a service area.

Using such inclusion criteria, researchers strive to achieve a balance between the specificity and the sensitivity of a medical service area definition. In other words, the researcher tries to define a medical service area whose residents exhibit a high degree of homogeneity (i.e., residents of the market area tend to visit the same hospital) while at the same time trying to select a medical service area that includes all of the patients of interest (i.e., all of the ZIP code areas that send patients to the study hospital). A medical service area that is too large would be extremely heterogeneous in terms of the utilization patterns of its residents, but would have a large number of patients; the latter characteristic is often desirable when calculating rates for comparisons. On the other hand, a medical service area that is too narrowly defined would have only a small number of patients, but would be extremely homogeneous in terms of the utilization patterns of its residents. In such a market area, dilution of the population by patients receiving care at institutions other than the one of interest would be relatively low.

Griffith (1972) and others have pointed out a number of difficulties with patient origin methodology. The definition of patient origin-based medical service areas is most difficult in urban areas where many hospitals are likely to draw patients from a single ZIP code (or other small) area. Likewise, when patients travel long distances for specialized care, the result is a geographic distribution of patients that is too sparse to draw a meaningful patient origin medical service area. Finally, the patient origin approach assumes that the distribution of patients among providers is stable over time within a fairly large geographic area. Such stability may not exist, particularly near the edges of market areas where market share is low. Diehr (1990) identifies several issues that must be considered when the patient origin method is used to define medical service areas. Her research indicates that the homogeneity of the size and age of the population used to calculate rates may strongly affect any hypothesis tests.

Medical service areas defined by the patient origin approach have been used successfully in descriptive, evaluative and, to some extent, planning research. Small area analysis is often used to describe variations in admission rates and is perhaps the most common descriptive application of patient origin techniques. Standards for the size of areas to examine and comparison methodologies have not yet been developed for small area analysis. Most commonly, small area studies have used variations and combinations of Griffith's measures of commitment and relevance to define medical service areas. Wright and Marlor (1990) point out that inclusion criteria used in past studies are often employed in subsequent studies with little conceptual justification, resulting in medical service areas that contain a substantial arbitrary element. Market share cutoffs used in prior research range from fifty to ninety percent, and the geographic scope of the medical service area is very sensitive to changes in these inclusion criteria (Goody, 1993b).

Griffith et al. (1981), Humphrey and Buechner (1992) and others have employed cluster analysis techniques to aggregate small areas. The primary objective of this technique is to group the smallest units together in clusters such that the variation in market share patterns within the clusters is minimized relative to the variation among the clusters. This technique has been applied with some frequency, but its validity is questionable. The clustering process requires a large degree of subjective judgment, and the resulting medical service areas will vary when different researchers create the clusters.

In summary, patient origin methods are ideal when a service area must be defined for a subpopulation or for a subgroup of diagnoses and when funding follows the individual. When selecting among patient origin techniques, researchers should use caution to ensure that the chosen technique examines the research question from the most appropriate perspective and that any violations of the underlying assumptions of the chosen technique are considered.

Selection of an Approach

As these descriptions indicate, the three methods of medical service area definition differ from each other in significant ways. The definition method used in a given research study can have a large impact on the researcher's findings. Therefore the choice of an appropriate medical service area definition method should be deliberate and informed. We have identified the following seven factors that should be considered in determining the appropriate definition method for a given study.

Criteria for the Selection of a Service Area Definition Technique

1. THE PURPOSE OF THE STUDY is the first important factor to consider. If the purpose is to analyze the economic exchange decisions of patients, then the geographic distance method would give the best result, all else being equal. If the medical service area will be used to define populations that are served by specific programs or providers, then the geopolitical boundary or patient origin methods would work better.

2. ECONOMIC AND ADMINISTRATIVE CHARACTERISTICS OF THE PROGRAMS INVOLVED should be considered. If the financing of services follows the individual, i.e., is based on individual eligibility, and services can be provided by either private or public providers, then the patient origin method may work best. If financing follows a program, the geopolitical or geographic distance method may yield the better medical service area definition.

3. ANALYTIC ADEQUACY (POWER) is an important consideration for any inferential study and predictive validity is essential for accurate forecasting. The three methods may behave very differently on these dimensions and the performance of each method should be considered before a final choice is made. Distance-based medical service areas have been more common in predictive studies. To maximize the power of a study we must trade off increases in power generated by defining medical service areas to include a large number of patients against decreases in power resulting from the inevitable dilution of the population of interest as the medical service areas increase in size.

4. MAJOR ISSUES RELATED TO BARRIERS TO ACCESS must be considered in the selection of a method for defining medical service areas. The validity of medical service areas that are based on distance measures may be influenced by the availability of public transportation and the presence of major road systems, mountains, lakes or rivers. Medical service areas that are defined by patient origin may not reflect recent shifts in markets, and their inclusion of charity/no pay regions will depend on such patients being treated administratively the same way as paying patients. If this is not consistently the case across institutions then the resulting variations in the medical service areas may influence the validity of the conclusions of a study.

5. THE STRUCTURE OF EXISTING REFERRAL PATTERNS is especially important to consider if a purpose of the study is to evaluate an innovation aimed at integrating care, improving access and utilization, or managing resource consumption. In such studies it would be desirable to use geopolitically defined medical service areas to reflect administrative/funding realities, or to use geographic distance to incorporate patient convenience preferences. Neither method will,

however, perform well if the decision on where to get care is made by referring physicians through well-established channels that do not coincide with distance criteria or geopolitical boundaries.

6. DIFFERENCES IN USE PATTERNS AMONG SUB-POPULATIONS should be considered when use patterns differ among patients of different age, race, income, socioeconomic level, or educational level. Each of the three methods should be assessed separately to clarify how expected differences in population use patterns would influence the validity of the medical service area's definition, given the purpose of the study.

7. DIFFERENCES IN USE PATTERNS ACROSS CLINICAL PROCEDURES must also be considered. Some clinical procedures may be termed "convenience goods," e.g., routine general care. Most patients will go to the nearest facility to get such interventions. Other procedures fall in the category of "shopping goods"; patients shop around until they find a price–feature combination that satisfies them, e.g., obstetrical deliveries. A third type of procedure may be classified as "specialty goods," e.g., coronary artery bypass graft operations. Generally, patients seek such procedures from recognized expert providers, often upon the advice of generalist providers.

Table 7-1 gives examples of predictive, descriptive and evaluative research studies that could employ each of the three medical service area definition methods.

Illustrations of Appropriate Applications of Medical Service Area Definition

Three examples of appropriate applications of medical service area definition to specific research questions are:

Example A: Site selection to maximize access for AIDS patients;

Example B: Determining the impact of public funding of prenatal care on rates of low birthweight; and

Example C: Determining the impact of hospital closure in rural areas on vulnerable Medicare sub-groups.

The criteria for selecting a method of medical service area definition for each example are discussed.

Table 7-1
Potential Applications of
Medical Service Area Definition Methods

	Planning/ Predictive	Descriptive	Evaluative
Geographic Distance Method	Does variation in utilization across medical service areas within a greater metropolitan area reflect imbalances of service capacity among those medical service areas? What potential reductions in patient travel time might be achieved with a more efficient distribution of facilities?	Do rates of specialized surgery decrease with increased geographic distance from a major teaching hospital?	Does the addition of a CCU to an existing hospital increase the rate of good cardiac case outcomes in the population within a thirty-mile radius of the hospital?
Geopolitical Method	Are public funds currently distributed in such a way that poor, high-risk patients in most counties have similar utilization patterns?	What are the differences in the rates of children with lead poisoning in states with strict automobile exhaust regulation and those using less strict criteria?	Does federal funding of demonstration projects for HIV prevention decrease state HIV infection rates compared to those noted in otherwise similar states without demonstration projects?
Patient Origin Method	Does hospital X serve a wide enough market area to justify continuing public funding to keep it open?	What are the surgical hospital admission rates for New Yorkers living in urban areas? In rural areas?	Does greater competition lead to higher hospital costs?

Example A

PURPOSE: SITE SELECTION TO MAXIMIZE ACCESS FOR AIDS
PATIENTS

1. PURPOSE OF STUDY: Find locations that maximize the utilization and minimize the cost of travel. Therefore select Geographic Distance (GD) approach.

2. ECONOMIC AND ADMINISTRATIVE CHARACTERISTICS OF THE PROGRAMS INVOLVED: The sources of funds and authority are mixed for such programs. This criterion is of little importance here.

3. ANALYTIC ADEQUACY (POWER): This type of project is predictive not inferential, so the issue of statistical power does not arise. Because we have few data available for predicting utilization by AIDS patients, a simple method of minimizing time and travel costs for patients would lead us toward the GD approach.

4. MAJOR ISSUES RELATED TO BARRIERS TO ACCESS: Indigent and minority patients have severe barriers to access to care in most communities. These sub-groups are also at high risk for HIV infection. The GD approach will allow us to define the medical service areas to specifically minimize the influence of these barriers to access if we weigh access by high-risk groups heavily in the medical service area formulation.

5. STRUCTURE OF EXISTING REFERRAL PATTERNS: Routine AIDS care for the majority of patients at this stage of the epidemic consists of primary care. Primary care decisions are generally made by patients or their families, who, in most cases would try to minimize travel time and cost. The GD assumptions fit well here.

6. DIFFERENCES IN USE PATTERNS AMONG SUB-POPULATIONS: There are major differences in use patterns among sub-

populations of AIDS patients. Many middle class patients purposely seek care outside their community to prevent information from 'leaking' about their HIV status. Poor and homeless AIDS patients seek the closest source that is willing to care for them. The most inclusive service area definition for wealthy patients is based on patient origin, but many poor and homeless patients could be excluded if this method were used. The geopolitically-defined medical service area fits neither the patients who travel outside of their community to seek care, nor those who seek care close to where they live. Thus, the GD method is the best choice based on this criterion.

7. DIFFERENCES IN USE PATTERNS ACROSS CLINICAL PROCEDURES: AIDS patients use different types of services during the course of the disease. Those in the late stages need more high-technology support and more specialist care. For this group the most appropriate medical service area definition would be that based on patient origin information. AIDS patients who are IV drug users may need Methadone support. For such patients, distance minimization is important. This criterion indicates that the analyst must decide on the relative importance of these two groups in the study.

APPROACH SELECTED:

Use geographic distance (GD) from patient to place of service. Rationale: This method meets the requirements of more of the seven criteria than do the alternative methods.

Example B

PURPOSE: TO DETERMINE THE IMPACT OF PUBLIC FUNDING OF PRENATAL CARE ON RATES OF LOW BIRTHWEIGHT (LBW)

1. PURPOSE OF STUDY: To determine if higher rates of funding for prevention of LBW result in lower rates of LBW births, *ceteris paribus.*

2. ECONOMIC AND ADMINISTRATIVE CHARACTERISTICS OF THE PROGRAMS INVOLVED: County Health Departments are the traditional providers of prenatal care for poor women. These facilities use federal, state, and local funds for programs, with the county as the most common base level of administrative authority. Increasingly, Medicaid pays for similar care and services are available through private providers. However, data on these services can be aggregated by county. Therefore select the geopolitical approach.

3. ANALYTIC ADEQUACY (POWER): This type of analysis requires the researcher to use statistical means of controlling for differences in risk of LBW. Most of the important control variables are available for county-level aggregations. It would be close to impossible to get information on community-level risk factors for distance-defined or patient origin-defined medical service areas.

4. MAJOR ISSUES RELATED TO BARRIERS TO ACCESS: High risk of LBW is correlated with minority, teenage and poverty status. Many teenage, poor, and minority women depend on public clinics in their county for care. This leads us towards the geopolitical approach.

5. STRUCTURE OF EXISTING REFERRAL PATTERNS: High-risk pregnant women often receive care at special regional clinics. They are, however, usually referred by local providers, and data on them may be allocated to their

[Example B, continued]

county of residence. Medical service area specification by the patient origin method would be the selection of choice for such women, and the geopolitical method would be the second best choice.

6. DIFFERENCES IN USE PATTERNS AMONG SUB-POPULATIONS: The use of publicly funded prenatal care is unequally distributed across communities and populations. Convenience and cost of care will affect a woman's utilization of care. This leads us to suggest medical service area definition by patient origin for self-pay or insured women, medical service area definition by geographic distance for women who get care in free clinics, and medical service area definition by the geopolitical method for women who seek care in county clinics.

7. DIFFERENCES IN USE PATTERNS ACROSS CLINICAL PROCEDURES: Prenatal care uses mainly low technology procedures, leading us to expect few differences across procedures. This criterion therefore provides little guidance for medical service area definition in the case of prenatal care.

APPROACH SELECTED:

Compare rates using geopolitically defined medical service area (counties). Rationale: Many of the data required are aggregated at the level of the county. The most consistent unit for administrative authority, reporting, and eligibility determination is the county.

Example C

PURPOSE: TO DETERMINE THE IMPACT OF HOSPITAL CLOSURE IN RURAL AREAS ON VULNERABLE MEDICARE SUB-GROUPS

1. PURPOSE OF STUDY: To determine whether local hospital access impacts the use and outcomes of care for Medicare patients with multiple diagnoses of psychiatric, alcohol and drug related problems. The patient origin approach is most closely linked to an individual institution's historical service area and is, therefore, the method of choice.

2. ECONOMIC AND ADMINISTRATIVE CHARACTERISTICS OF THE PROGRAMS INVOLVED: Medicare patients can receive care anywhere, and the program is nationally administered. Therefore, this criteria provides no specific guidance for specifying medical service areas.

3. ANALYTIC ADEQUACY (POWER): The statistical power in this study is maximized if the medical service areas are defined so that they have the greatest number of Medicare eligibles and the least dilution of this population by Medicare patients who receive care in a competing hospital. Of the three methods, the patient origin method is the only one that allows the researcher to account for sensitivity and specificity as they affect statistical power while defining market areas. Therefore, select the patient origin approach.

4. MAJOR ISSUES RELATED TO BARRIERS TO ACCESS: Medicare patients who need hospitalization for psychiatric, alcohol, and drug related conditions can get care anywhere—they are not limited by any geopolitical boundaries. They would be expected to follow the local hospital market pattern in seeking care. Likewise, hospital closure would be expected to have an impact on those people who visited the hospital prior to closure. Therefore, the patient origin approach is the most appropriate for this study.

[Example C, continued]

5. STRUCTURE OF EXISTING REFERRAL PATTERNS: Treatment decisions are made by patients and their providers. Referral patterns are not limited by funding or other political factors. Patients, then, can be treated at a local or a distant hospital. As a result, referral patterns are not likely to consistently follow any geopolitical or geographical boundaries. The patient origin method defines market areas that reflect what can be relatively unpredictable referral patterns.

6. DIFFERENCES IN USE PATTERNS AMONG SUB-POPULATIONS: are specific for Medicare patients and vary by diagnosis within this group. Market area specification should therefore be based on Medicare data on patient origin for psychiatric, alcohol, and drug use related DRGs. The patient origin method is unique because it enables the researcher to define population-specific and diagnosis-specific market areas.

7. DIFFERENCES IN USE PATTERNS ACROSS CLINICAL PROCEDURES: There would be minimal variation in use patterns across procedures for this group of diagnoses. This criterion is not very useful for guiding market area definition in the case of Medicare alcohol, drug and psychiatric related hospitalizations.

APPROACH SELECTED:

Use patient origin data to aggregate ZIP codes by the DRG market share for the hospitals of interest. Rationale: Individual-level data are available across geopolitical boundaries, and this approach allows for the maximization of statistical power.

▷ P O I N T
▷ OF DEPARTURE

Hospital Closure and Access
to Hospital Services
John Lowe

The issue of hospital closure is very important to rural and urban communities. The last decade has seen a dramatic rise in the number of total closings and rural communities have been especially hard hit. In 1991, 45 hospitals closed and 29 of them were in rural areas. Closure of any hospital may place strain on the remaining facilities serving the poor and create gaps in access to hospital services for urban and rural patient populations. Understanding the effects of hospital closure on populations is difficult since patient use behaviors do not follow set patterns.

This Point of Departure describes a methodology for estimating changes in hospital patient volumes in an urban hospital market as a result of one or more hospital closures. The choice of an urban example was dictated by the availability of data but the technique applied here can be used in rural and cross-regional studies. The method used here, the *gravity model*, is useful for detecting hospitals that may be most affected by the closure of selected facilities. By extending the model and tying it to other patterns of utilization, the impact of hospital closure on patient populations in specific geographic areas can also be examined.

The Gravity Model

Gravity models are representative of spatial interaction approaches to understanding "flows" in a system. These include commuter flows in transportation systems, dollar flows in international trade, and flows of people in interstate migration. Gravity models have been used in health care to describe hospital flows in a rural market (Meade, 1974), optimize hospital facility location decisions (Mayhew, Gibberd & Hall, 1986), and analyze the effects of inner city hospital closures (McLafferty, 1988). The gravity model is appropriate for analyzing aggregate patient flows in a regional hospital market since they are conveniently estimated with aggregate data and may provide results more easily transferable to other locations.

Over the last two decades the multinomial Logit[1] model has emerged as a primary method for modeling hospital choice. The Logit model and the gravity model are similar in many respects. The Logit model is applicable where there is a choice to use or not use a particular facility. For example, Logit models can describe the probability of a person at one location choosing a hospital at another location *and* the probability of that hospital being chosen by the person. In essence the person may or may not choose a particular hospital and the model can assign a probability to that. At the same time the model can calculate the probability of the hospital being chosen by a person from a particular place. Combining these two models yields the gravity model. What is more, this gravity model uniquely describes the two Logit models.

Model Formulation

The application described here uses a generalized gravity model to estimate changes in patient volumes in an urban

[1]Logit is essentially a multiple regression model where the values of the dependent variable are categorical (e.g., high/low; 200-150, 149-100, 99-50, 49-0) rather than continuous (e.g., 0, 1, 2, 3, ..., ∞).

hospital market as a result of multiple hospital closures. The model is of the form:

(1) $T_{ij} = E(N_{ij}) = A(i)B(j)F(c_{ij})$ where:

T_{ij} =   predicted flow of patients from zone of residence i to hospital destination j. A zone of residence is usually a small area such as a minor civil division, or ZIP code for rural areas.

$A(i)$ =   a composite measure of "propulsiveness" for hospital trips at origin i. This is based on the ability of people in the area to use the hospital in the target area.

$B(j)$ =   a composite measure of "attractiveness" of hospital j which is based upon factors that might cause people to choose this hospital over others; these are "market" variables.

$F(c_{ij})$ = a composite of measures of separation between the origin and the destination. This is usually measured in terms of travel times or distance.

In order to apply the model, an algebraic form for the separation factors, $F(c_{ij})$, is needed. The form that is used in this application is:

(2) $F(c_{ij}^{k}) = \exp[0'c_{ij}^{k}]$

where c_{ij} represents a vector of k measures of separation or distance and $0' = (0_1 \ldots 0_k)$ is a vector of parameters to be estimated using maximum likelihood or least squares procedures.

Separation Factors

A key component of the gravity model is the specification of the distance or separation factor(s). Separation measures used in this application are travel time between ZIP code centroid and hospital, and a measure of non-spatial distance representing socioeconomic "distance" between residents of a certain ZIP code and a hospital. The particular specification of nonspatial separation employed in an analysis of spatial separation in the Chicago examples is given by:

$$c_{ij} = \log\left[\sum_{M=1}^{M} \sqrt{p_i^{(m)}} \sqrt{q_j^{(m)}}\right]$$

then:

$$\exp[c_{ij}] = \begin{cases} 1 & \text{Match Perfect} \\ 0 & \text{No Match} \end{cases}$$

where:

$p_i =$ the proportion of payer sources in each of M payer categories of persons residing in i; and

$q_j =$ the proportion of payer sources in each category for services offered by hospital j.

The resulting measure is an index of the degree of "match" in the profile of payer categories (i.e., Medicare, Medicaid, commercial insurance and self-pay) for patients in each ZIP code and for the patient mix at each hospital.

Origin and Destination Factors

The generalized gravity model incorporates the characteristics of the hospitals into the destination–attractiveness factors (B_j's) and characteristics of the origin zones into origin–propulsiveness (A_i's) factors. In the generalized model, the origin and destination factors are estimated by the model. The Deming-Stephan Furness procedure solves for these factors iteratively, starting with any positive $B(j)$, with solutions converging on a single value. Earlier efforts to set them as *a priori* functions led to inconsistencies (e.g., in the studies of migration $A(i)$ and $B(j)$ would be set as functions of populations of zones i and j).

Case Study: Hospital Closures in Chicago, Illinois

The six-county Chicago Metropolitan Area is defined as the market area. The 92 short-term, acute care hospitals in this area receive at least 88% of their patient load from these six counties, with 90 hospitals deriving over 95% of their patients from there.

The market is divided into 250 postal ZIP code origin zones. Post office box, commercial ZIP codes and other ZIP codes not defining a specific geographic area were eliminated from the sample. Over 98% of the hospital trips made by residents of these ZIP codes were made to hospitals in the study area.

The results illustrated in the map of the Chicago region in Figure 7-6 are based on a model using square root of travel time and payer match as the measures of separation. The model is calibrated using 1987 patient discharge data, i.e., the model is run first using historical data. Origin, destination and separation values are obtained from the model.

Between 1987 and 1990 six inner city hospitals in the Chicago market closed. The gravity model obtained above is re-estimated using the same total number of hospital trips from all ZIP codes for 1987 (N_{i+}), the same separation factor (F_{ij}) and the same destination factors (B_j's) for all hospitals, except the closed hospitals. The destination factors for the closed hospitals are set equal to zero, since closed facilities "attract" no patients.

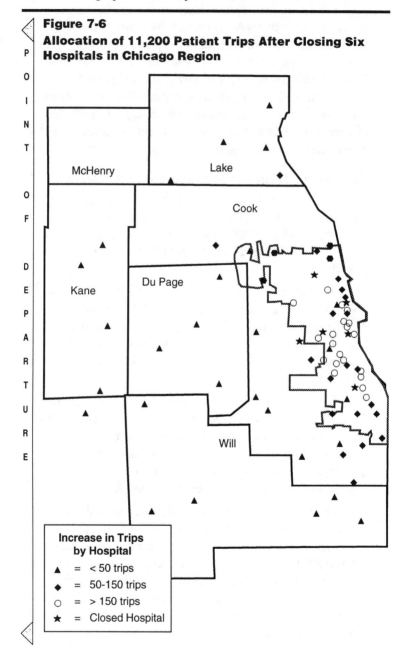

Figure 7-6
Allocation of 11,200 Patient Trips After Closing Six Hospitals in Chicago Region

The model re-allocates the 11,200 patient trips which would have gone to the closed facilities to the remaining hospitals in the system. Based on the separation measures, we would expect hospitals relatively close to the closed hospitals and which treat a somewhat similar patient mix in terms of payer sources to receive a larger share of these patient trips. These results are shown graphically in Figure 7-6.

Once the anticipated new hospital destinations for patients from each ZIP code are obtained from the gravity model, an analysis of potential changes in patients' access to hospital services can be conducted. The new hospital destinations for the population can be translated into average travel times based on each ZIP code. The travel times for the new ZIP code–hospital combinations can be compared to the original results to see if there are changes in total access time. If each ZIP code or smaller division can be assigned proxy income levels, then the model can describe changes in access for the poor versus the non-poor.

This model provides a statistical basis for estimating patient flows that are redirected following a reduction in health care resources (hospital closure in this case). However, in using this model the researcher should be cognizant of the factors it does not incorporate, such as the influence of marketing efforts, patient perceptions of quality of care, and physician referral patterns.

POINT OF DEPARTURE

Chapter 8

Contagious Diseases

Point of Departure:
Adjustment of Tuberculosis Incidence Rates

Introduction

Knowing how contagious diseases are distributed and how they diffuse across space and time is important for prevention and timely intervention and control. Contagious diseases, with the possible exception of influenza, drew less and less attention in the medical care system because of their perceived diminishing incidence and prevalence and the expanded use of vaccines and therapies that could reduce their effects. We now face an emerging threat from infectious diseases. The agents that cause diseases thought to be brought under control like gonorrhea and malaria have grown resistant to drugs that once contained them. New disease agents threaten to change in such a way as to cross from animal into human populations; indeed some hypothesize that this is the origin of infectious retroviruses. In the last two decades these changes threaten to introduce a new era where infectious diseases regain their place as a major killer and crippler.

The decline of some infectious diseases cannot be ascribed to medical interventions; we really can't explain the decline of scarlet fever in general and leprosy in Europe, or why tuberculosis became less of a problem even before antibiotics were introduced. Rene Dubos (1965) attributed much of the decline of contagious disease to changes in societal behavior, population distribution and mobility, and the built environment to which people are adapting. Geography can take into consideration this built environment and the social structure of human settlement and migration as it tracks the movement of disease through space and time.

This chapter gives examples of how this can be done, first by offering definitions of different types of diffusion, then describing studies of diffusion and the development of models to predict diffusion. This overview of diffusion processes is followed by two examples that illustrate how the spread of AIDS and tuberculosis can be examined and predicted using geographic techniques.

Disease Diffusion

Diffusion is the movement of ideas, innovations, or just about anything—contagious diseases in this case—through space and time. In many respects, spatial diffusion manifests itself in ways that are analogous to the effects of waves on the shoreline or the movement of weather fronts as seen on weather maps. From such analogies, diffusion is often described in terms of "diffusion waves" or "clinical fronts."

Diffusion in its general sense implies movement in all directions. However, in most instances, elements of the cultural and physical environment interact to produce channels for or barriers to a given disease. Four major types of diffusion have been identified: expansion, contagious, hierarchical, and relocation. *Expansion diffusion* is the gradual spread of a disease outward from a center of concentration in such a way that both the number of people and the area affected by the disease increase from the epicenter or initial case observance. *Contagious diffusion* is similar to expansion diffusion in that it spreads through a population; the term is more specific because it implies direct person-to-person contact or local transmission or contiguity effects. *Hierarchical diffusion* is the movement of a disease through levels or ranks of a system. For example, a disease could move from urban to rural places by first affecting residents in New York City (a very large city), then Pittsburgh, Pennsylvania (a moderate size city), and finally Butler (a small, rural town outside of Pittsburgh). In a similar manner, certain diseases can also filter down (or up) through different social or income classes. In *relocation diffusion*, disease spreads from one initial center to more distant locations through long-distance inter-action such as the movement of people from one place to another. This could happen through migration (individuals moving from one place to another) that introduces a disease common to the place of origin but uncommon to the destination site. Other diffusion processes have been observed where contagious diseases spread through more than one of these diffusion processes. The four diffusion processes identified above refer to movement through space; adding the dimension of time completes the description of diffusion and moves the analysis away from static snapshots of distribution. The use of space and time in combination is essential to an understanding of the process of diffusion.

Diffusion processes do not operate in a vacuum, and the direction and degree of penetration of a given disease is often a function of the structure of biological and physical systems across which a disease spreads. These systems can be facilitators or barriers to the spread of disease. Barriers exist in three basic types: absorbing, reflecting, and permeable. An *absorbing barrier* stops or attenuates (weakens) diffusion to the extent that a disease is unable to reach across or beyond a barrier. A *reflecting barrier* reflects the diffusion wave, acting to channel and/or strengthen the movement of a disease along certain pathways. With a *permeable barrier* the diffusion of a disease is able to penetrate the barrier although the strength of the diffusion wave is weakened to some degree. All of these types of barriers can be further differentiated as either physical or cultural in nature. Some examples of physical barriers are mountains, deserts, swamps, lakes, and oceans. Cultural barriers are often the product of differences in language, religion, or political philosophy.

Medical geographers and others have frequently used the concepts of spatial diffusion to examine the movement of disease and health care innovations through time and space. Four examples of diffusion analysis by geographers folllow:

- Baker (1979) found the diffusion of computerized axial tomography (CT scanners) to be hierarchical according to hospital size as measured by number of beds.

- Adesina (1984) examined how cholera diffused outside Ibadan City (dominant urban center of the former Western State of Nigeria) during the 1971 epidemic. The diffusion of cholera was hierarchical when towns were distinguished from villages: towns, with a larger population base than the villages, all confronted the cholera epidemic before the villages. However, a positive significant correlation was found between a town's distance from Ibadan and the week of onset of cholera at the town, suggesting that the spread of cholera outside Ibadan was more a function of distance decay (i.e., towns further from Ibadan were affected by the epidemic later than were closer towns). The epidemic emanating outward from Ibadan was observed to be more a product of contagious and expansion diffusion rather than hierarchical diffusion.

- Patterson and Pyle (1983) found that the spread of influenza in sub-Saharan Africa during the 1918-1919 pandemic operated through relocation and expansion diffusion. Influenza skipped along the coast of West Africa via shipping contacts (a form of relocation diffusion) from Freetown, Sierra Leone, north to Dakar (Senegal) and south and then east to Accra (Ghana), Lagos (Nigeria), and Douala (Cameroon). From these coastal ports, influenza spread along colonial transport networks to the interior hinterlands of the respective ports. The movement of influenza from coastal to interior routes set up a "clinical front" advancing towards French Equatorial Africa (Central African Republic).

- Cliff, Haggett and Stroup (1992) analyzed the geographic structure of the measles epidemic in the northeastern United States. The most striking feature of this epidemic was the dominance of the contagious diffusion process or local transmission of the disease. However, interstate bonds were observed, suggesting the operation of both hierarchical and expansion diffusion processes as well.

Geographical techniques used in modeling diffusion and in designing community vaccination or other interventions and controls have also been utilized to study a variety of vector-borne and contagious diseases (Cliff & Haggett, 1988). (Vectors are carriers of disease—ticks, mosquitoes, liver flukes. Contagious processes are usually the direct transfer of a disease agent—bacteria, virus, parasite—from victim to victim.) These techniques have recently been developed further and used to model the diffusion of measles and influenza (Cliff, Haggett & Ord, 1986; Pyle, 1986). Thomas (1992) has described in detail various mathematical and stochastic models for describing infectious disease as a geomedical system, including transmission of tuberculosis and AIDS. Modeling these diffusion processes can help control or eliminate a contagious disease in a population.

In the United States, Acquired Immunodeficiency Syndrome (AIDS) and Tuberculosis (TB) are current epidemics of increasing public health concern. Decisions about financing the prevention and treatment of these diseases frequently fall to government officials who must allocate limited resources based on the most current information available. In this chapter, we will demonstrate some geographic techniques that may be used to address problems of resource allocation and to answer questions frequently asked about AIDS and TB.

Acquired Immunodeficiency Syndrome (AIDS)

Background

As of September 1993, there were over 339,250 cases of AIDS reported to the Centers for Disease Control and Prevention, and almost 20 percent or 62,102 of these were reported as new cases in 1992 alone (CDC, 1993). The CDC has estimated in 1990 that 1 to 1.5 million Americans were infected with the human immunodeficiency virus (HIV). Ongoing surveillance of reported AIDS cases has shown that the initial, major epicenters in New York, California and Florida are contributing smaller percentages of new cases as the epidemic spreads to other areas of the United States (CDC, 1991a).

AIDS has become an increasingly important problem in the small towns and rural areas of America (Davis & Stapleton, 1991; Verghese, Berk & Sarubbi, 1989). Recent studies have found a disproportionately high HIV seroprevalence in the southern United States among disadvantaged adolescents (St. Louis et al., 1991), migrant farmers (CDC, 1988), and military recruits (Gardner et al., 1989). The federal government allocates its HIV/AIDS funds based upon the number of AIDS cases diagnosed in each state. A concern that health care resources in rural communities may not be adequate to meet the needs of persons with AIDS has emerged with the diffusion of new AIDS cases from predominantly urban to more rural areas. Given the growing AIDS burden, states must determine how best to allocate resources for HIV/AIDS education, prevention, and medical care.

Examining the Diffusion of AIDS

Geographic analysis can help us answer specific questions about AIDS to give us direction in meeting the public health challenges presented by this disease: How has the epidemic changed over time? How has it spread through the settlement pattern, demographic groups, and spatial structure of the population? Has AIDS diffused into rural areas of the US? Has AIDS diffused into rural areas in my state? Where should the State provide HIV/AIDS health services?

We first examine how the AIDS epidemic has changed over time. AIDS has spread worldwide but followed different paths and afflicted various people (Shannon, Pyle & Bashshur, 1991). In some places, it is heterosexually transmitted and both sexes are equally afflicted. In others the principal transmission is through homosexuals. It can be introduced through drug abuse, and crosses rapidly into commercial prostitution. It spreads along highways via truckers and labor migration, and in other places it has spread through a contaminated blood supply. In the United States, the rate of increase of AIDS is currently most rapid among the teenage sexual partners of intravenous drug abusers. In 1981, after early reports of *Pneumocystis carinii* pneumonia, Kaposi's sarcoma, and other opportunistic infections in young homosexual men in Los Angeles, New York City, and San Francisco, the CDC began collecting information on all cases of what is now termed the Acquired Immunodeficiency Syndrome. By 1985, all states had regulations requiring physicians and other health care providers to report AIDS cases directly to their state or local health department. These health departments then shared their respective reports with CDC, which produces the national AIDS surveillance data set.

Karon and Berkelman (1991) at CDC recently examined the geographic and ethnic diversity of AIDS incidence trends in homosexual and bisexual men in the United States from 1983 through 1990 using the national AIDS surveillance data set. Their primary method for examining AIDS incidence trends was visual. They plotted adjusted (because of reporting delays) AIDS incidence along with smoothed curves obtained from a local weighted average of adjusted incidence for January of 1983 through September of 1990 (Figure 8-1). Although these surveillance data show a plateau or near plateau in AIDS incidence (cases diagnosed per calendar quarter) in New York, San Francisco, and Los Angeles, and in many other large Metropolitan Statistical Areas (MSAs) with a population of at least 1 million, no slowing in the rate of growth of incidence was found in rural and smaller metropolitan areas of the United States. The incidence of AIDS among gay and bisexual men has continued to increase linearly through 1990 in rural areas

Figure 8-1

AIDS incidence in men reporting homosexual and bisexual contact and not using IV drugs in the United States, 1983-1990, by size of Metropolitan Statistical Area of residence, based on cases reported through March 1991.

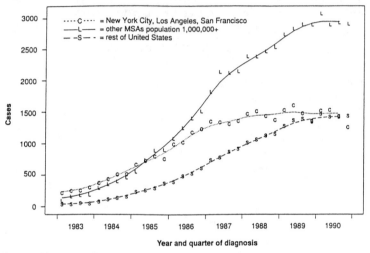

Year and quarter of diagnosis

Source: Karon and Berkelman, p. 1182.

(population <50,000) and small MSAs (population <1 million) as compared with larger MSAs (population >1,000,000).

The spatial analysis of incidence trends requires adjustment of the directly calculated rates to account for variations in the comparison populations. Two methods of adjustment or standardization are presented in the Point of Departure accompanying this chapter.

The number of diagnosed AIDS cases increased an estimated ten percent from 1990 to 1991 (CDC, 1991a). Larger proportionate increases occurred among women compared with men and among blacks and Hispanics compared with non-Hispanic whites. Among US regions, the South reported the highest number of cases as well as the greatest proportionate increase in cases from 1990-1991. In the Northeast, the annual number of diagnosed cases among homo-

Figure 8-2

**AIDS cases among persons reporting heterosexual contact
with persons with or at high risk for HIV infection*, by
region† and year of diagnosis: United States, 1988-1991§**

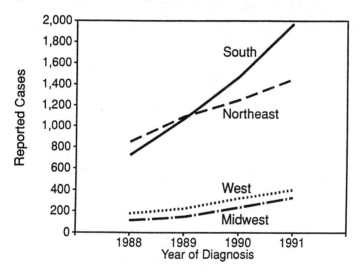

*Adjusted for reporting delays.

†South comprises the South Atlantic, East South Central, and West South Central
regions; Northeast comprises the New England and Middle Atlantic Regions;
West comprises the Mountain and Pacific regions; and Midwest comprises the
East North Central and West North Central regions.

§Each group analyzed includes a percentage of persons with no identified risk
(NIR) that belong to the same geographic categories. The redistribution of NIR
cases is based on sex- and race/ethnicity-specific exposure category distributions of cases diagnosed from 1984 through 1988 that were initially assigned to
NIR category but were subsequently reclassified.

Source: Centers for Disease Control. *MMWR* 1992;41: p. 67.

sexual and bisexual men remained relatively stable or decreased.
During 1988-1991, the highest number of cases and the most rapid
increase in cases occurred in the South among homosexual and
bisexual men. Although cases among persons exposed to HIV
through heterosexual contact increased in all regions, the South
reported the highest number of such cases in 1991 and the most rapid
increase in cases during the period 1988-1991 (Figure 8-2).

Figure 8-3

AIDS indence in men reporting homosexual or bisexual contact and not using IV drugs while living in the New York City Metropolitan Statistical Area, 1983-1990, based on cases reported through March 1991

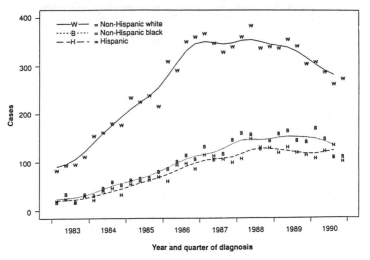

Source: Karon and Berkelman, p. 1183.

We next focus our examination of the AIDS epidemic on the extent to which the disease has diffused into rural areas within states across the US. Although the CDC does not regularly release its entire national AIDS surveillance data set, the Division of HIV/ AIDS (National Center for Infectious Disease, Centers for Disease Control and Prevention) biannually creates the AIDS Public Information Data Set, which contains data extracted from CDC's national AIDS surveillance data set. Using this data set, which is provided free of charge by the CDC, local government officials and public health researchers can answer questions concerning the trends in AIDS incidence in their area. Unfortunately for researchers, but in order to protect patient confidentiality, the public information data set contains only information on region of residence. For this reason, only the CDC, with its larger national AIDS data set, is capable of examining AIDS incidence in rural areas in any particular state. Although Karon and Berkelman (1991), at the CDC, were able to compare AIDS incidence by race in a particular city, similar analyses could be done using cases from all northeastern MSAs (Figure 8-3). By restricting data on AIDS incidence to those cases reported from non-MSA areas, policy makers could determine the trends in AIDS incidence for rural areas and use these findings to help determine how to direct continuing efforts to minimize the risks of transmission of HIV. Were data on residence at the time of infection with AIDS available by county, city, or ZIP code, our understanding of the burden of HIV disease in specific communities would be even greater.

To determine whether AIDS has diffused into rural areas and to answer the question of where a state should place HIV/AIDS health services, one might first determine where patients with HIV/AIDS are living. The CDC provides data on the number of AIDS cases reported both by state and by MSA with populations greater than 500,000, based on where patients were living when they were diagnosed with AIDS. Clearly this does not yield enough detail to determine where patients are currently living and where health services are most needed. Many state health departments also have data on place of residence for all cases of AIDS reported within that state, and will provide interested parties with tallies of number of patients reported with AIDS per county. Some states also have mandatory reporting of HIV seropositivity, producing similar data for people with HIV prior to an AIDS diagnosis. The reluctance of the CDC and some states to release detailed information results from concerns about protecting confidentiality. For purposes of mapping and other geographic analyses, however, detail(s) on age, sex, ethnicity, income, or other socioeconomic descriptors that could help identify individuals are not needed. Most states will provide researchers with incidence rates at the county level. However, at this scale of analysis important patterns can be masked when analyzing utilization or mobility pathways of afflicted inidividuals if a study is restricted to a single state or fails to take into account regular commuting patterns or travel to other counties where exposure risk is markedly higher.

Another potential source of information about where HIV-infected persons live is from hospitals and health care centers where many HIV-infected patients receive services. Cohn et al. (1992) surveyed all HIV-infected patients seen at the UNC Hospitals over a four-month period in 1990. They obtained a ten-year residential history, including where people thought they became HIV-infected and where their families lived.

In the Cohn et al. study, distance measures were calculated with town name as a reference point to determine latitude and longitude coordinates using the US Geological Survey of Named and Populated Places (US Geological Survey, 1988). Population size of towns was obtained from the 1990 Census of Population and Housing (US Bureau of the Census, 1991). There are several ways to calculate distance measures depending on the data available and the size of the population. By determining the latitude and longitude coordinates of places, distance can be directly calculated using geometric equations. Microcomputer mapping programs are available (e.g., Tactician®, Atlas Pro®, GeoQuery®, MapInfo®), most of which can set home base coordinates and draw radii around points to determine not only distances, but also what lies within a designated radius around a point (e.g. hospital, patient).

This information was then used to plan for the provision of convenient, accessible health care for HIV-infected patients by comparing where they live with where they were going for the treatment of their disease. Using current town of residence, Cohn et al. determined the percent of patients living in metropolitan and nonmetropolitan counties as well as the percent living in towns of fewer than 50,000 persons. Of 325 HIV-infected patients who completed surveys, a third (32%) lived in counties designated as nonmetropolitan, and over half (56%) lived in towns with a population of greater than 50,000 (Figure 8-4). Of the total in both metro and nonmetro counties, 32 percent lived in towns of less than 10,000 population. Although the data presented in Figure 8-4 were obtained from one referral hospital in the center of the state, several conclusions could be drawn if they represented the entire popula-

Figure 8-4 **Distribution within North Carolina by County of Residence of HIV-Infected Patients Treated at University of North Carolina Hospitals Clinics**

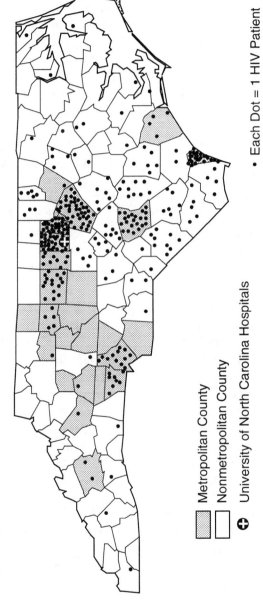

Metropolitan County
Nonmetropolitan County
✪ University of North Carolina Hospitals

• Each Dot = 1 HIV Patient

Dots are distributed randomly within county boundaries. N = 312.

tion with AIDS: 1) most patients reside in metropolitan counties; 2) patients travel long distances to be seen, 78 miles on average (range 0-561 miles); 3) a large concentration of patients travel over 135 miles from New Hanover County, a county on the southeastern coast of North Carolina. Using this map of the distribution of patients, a logical choice for locating new (or improved) health services would be in Wilmington, the town within New Hanover County with the largest number of HIV-infected patients. The HIV-infected population is apparently bypassing local hospitals. Perhaps there is a need for a specialized clinic which caters to AIDS patients, is sensitive and responsive to their needs, and will accept Medicaid. Perhaps there is a need to recruit a physician specializing in infectious disease who is interested and willing to care for AIDS patients, or to secure additional AIDS health care funds from the state or from the private sector (e.g., home care agencies). Additional studies would be necessary to explain why patients with HIV bypass their local hospital to be seen in a hospital 135 miles distant from their place of residence.

Another approach to understanding the diffusion of AIDS in North Carolina was taken by Pyle and Furuseth (1992), who found that HIV infection and AIDS became "seeded" in some counties of North Carolina between 1985 and 1987. They present a model of AIDS incidence in North Carolina in relation to settlement morphology. Their analysis observes the hierarchical spread of AIDS, first to the predominant metropolitan counties of Mecklenburg and Wake and then through the second-order metropolitan counties of the Piedmont Urban Crescent (i.e., counties with connection to interstate highways I-77, I-85, and I-40 between Charlotte and Raleigh) as a "second wave." In 1989, the hierarchical diffusion process filtered to the rural counties of eastern North Carolina. In addition to hierarchical diffusion, AIDS continues to be spread outward from nodal areas of infection such as Charlotte through contagious and expansion diffusion. There is a strong decrease in AIDS incidence rates with increasing distance from Charlotte; this is an indication that AIDS is diffusing as both an expansion and contagious process on the intra-metropolitan scale. However, on

Figure 8-5a **AIDS in North Carolina, 1990**

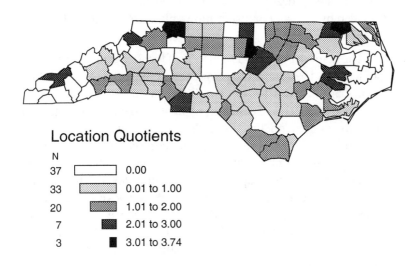

Location Quotients

N		
37		0.00
33		0.01 to 1.00
20		1.01 to 2.00
7		2.01 to 3.00
3		3.01 to 3.74

Figure 8-5b **AIDS in North Carolina, 1990**

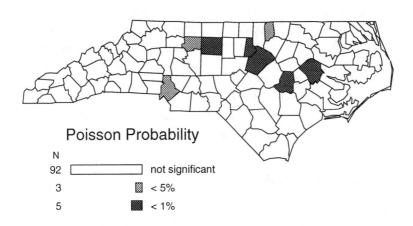

Poisson Probability

N		
92		not significant
3		< 5%
5		< 1%

Source: Dy CA. The Geography of AIDS in North Carolina. Unpublished honors essay, Department of Geography, University of North Carolina, 1991.

the inter-metropolitan scale, hierarchical diffusion dominates in the transmission of HIV and AIDS. In addition to providing insight into the diffusion process as it has occurred in the state, the model provided by Pyle and Furuseth allows planners to predict the future spread of the disease.

The maps in Figure 8-5a and 8-5b of location quotients of AIDS incidence in 1990 show the geography of the diffusion of AIDS in North Carolina (Dy, 1991). These maps were part of a thesis that examined the effects of distance, population size, and the interstate highway system on the disease's spread, using the analytical methodology of measuring spatial autocorrelation, which tests the probability that a rate in one place is affected by the rate in an adjacent place. The maps show the county-level pattern, using location quotients (see Chapters 3 and 5) and counties where incidence is higher than could occur by chance according to a Poisson (small number) distribution. Display options such as these are useful descriptive tools that are available to analysts, researchers, and planners.

These analyses illustrate the geographic aspects of the AIDS epidemic and help describe the increasing diversity of persons affected by the epidemic. Persons with AIDS reflect the larger population of HIV-infected persons who are asymptomatic or have other HIV-associated diseases. Trends in AIDS incidence show that there are no geographic barriers to the disease; our responses need to accept this and make access to care possible by targeting those places with growing numbers of cases. A similar examination of tuberculosis is provided in the next section, which discusses various options for examining the diffusion of another kind of disease process.

Mycobacterium Tuberculosis (TB)

Background

Since 1985, there has been a resurgence of TB in the United States. The disease, which was a leading killer at the beginning of this century, has begun to thrive once again, with 26,673 new cases reported in 1992 (CDC, 1993). As in the past, when tuberculosis was the scourge of the poor and the urban working masses, the new tuberculosis is once again the bane of the poorest sectors of society. The population subgroups hit hardest by the new wave of tuberculosis are the disenfranchised. Economic hardship and social dislocation combined with a dismantling of the public health infrastructure over the last decade or so have created the conditions for a resurgence of this disease.

Examining the Diffusion of TB

Similar to the case of AIDS, geographic analysis can be used to address questions related to tuberculosis and provide direction in meeting the challenges in health services delivery presented by this disease. We find ourselves asking questions such as: How has the TB epidemic changed over time? How has TB affected rural areas? What is the role played by farm workers in the new tuberculosis? Where should TB health services be concentrated? These questions are addressed as we examine the diffusion of tuberculosis.

Tuberculosis—once so prevalent in the Southeast that its treatment in asylums and rest homes influenced the development of Asheville, North Carolina, and other mountain towns and sandhills resorts—has been thought for several decades to be "conquered." After declining in incidence for most of the twentieth century, tuberculosis seemed to be disappearing as a result of both the availability after World War II of powerful new antibiotics to render people non-infective, even cured, and x-ray technology to diagnose new cases in screening programs. Unlike many other countries in the world, the United States never went into wholesale vaccination with BCG as a useful though not total preventative for TB, mainly because our incidence rate was brought so low that screening people with skin tests to detect exposure to the tubercle bacilli was more cost-effective. Tuberculosis seemed to have been a problem mainly of relapse among elderly people and other former patients undergoing stress. It was also a public health concern that, although persons with active TB were quarantined by the US Immigration and Naturalization service and active cases were not admitted, illegal immigrants were sometimes infective and were not detected by the public schools, large company employment, or other conventional screening situations. Still, the incidence was so low and the problem seemed so demographically limited that funding, screening, and active detection and treatment were greatly curtailed.

The emergence of antibiotic-resistant strains, the difficulty of keeping people non-infective if they do not continue a long regime of medicine, shortcomings and funding of community support and surveillance of that treatment regime, declining conditions of poor housing, poor nutrition, as well as immunological susceptibility are combining to produce a public health emergency. The population subgroups hardest hit by the new wave of tuberculosis are African-Americans, Hispanics, the homeless, alcoholics, the HIV-infected, the institutionalized (e.g., prisoners and nursing home residents), illegal immigrants from countries with a high prevalence of TB, and the poor in general.

The resurgence of TB is not just an urban problem. While the majority of those at high risk for TB live in urban areas, rural areas have not been exempt from an increase in TB cases. This time around, TB is reaching into rural areas not only through the poor in general, but specifically through itinerant agricultural workers who harvest the crops on farms in rural areas—migrant workers. This disease clearly spreads by both the contagious and expansion diffusion processes.

A majority of the migrant workers in the United States are of Hispanic origin, immigrants from countries with high rates of TB, or African-Americans who have higher rates of TB than the white population (NC Department of Labor, 1992; Migrant Health Task Force, 1991; Ciesielski et al., 1991). Living and working conditions for migrant workers are among the poorest of any occupation. An annual income of less than $12,500 for a family of four is the standard for measuring poverty in the United States. Migrant workers in 1989 had a mean annual income of $5,667 (Migrant Health Task Force, 1991). Poor sanitation facilities at home and at work, constant exposure to the chemical hazards of fertilizers and pesticides in the fields, and an inability to communicate adequately or be understood by medical workers they do see render migrant workers vulnerable to the effects of a wide array of infectious diseases and chronic conditions.

Ciesielski et al. (1991) examined TB among North Carolina migrant workers. North Carolina has the fifth highest number of migrant farm workers in the United States and employs the largest number of farm workers of any of the Eastern states (Migrant Health Task Force, 1991). Eighty-eight percent of migrant workers in the state are primarily Spanish-speaking (Migrant Health Task Force, 1991). In this tuberculosis study, migrant farm workers in 31 camps in five counties were randomly sampled for TB infection (Ciesielski et al., 1991). Two percent of the sample had active cases of tuberculosis with 0.47 percent occurring among Hispanics and 3.6 percent occurring among African-Americans—the latter case rate being more than 3,000 times the national case rate and seven times the Hispanic rate (Ciesielski et al., 1991). Despite the presence of migrant workers who were immigrants from countries with a high prevalence of TB, Ciesielski and his colleagues found that the most important source of TB was from US-born migrant workers (1991). A significant number of African-American migrant workers reported being recruited to farm work from homeless shelters, soup kitchens, and alcohol rehabilitation centers—environments identified as conducive to the spread of tuberculosis. There was a positive correlation between years in farm work and tuberculosis infection, demonstrating that for farm workers, TB is an occupational disease (Ciesielski et al., 1991).

The findings of the Ciesielski et al. study suggest that the geography of tuberculosis is important since migrant labor is tied to specific crops. Examining the geography of the disease could help in targeting special outreach public health programs specifically designed to reach migrant farm workers. Many of these workers have contacts with local communities and go back and forth between the farms and these areas. In addition, many immigrant farm workers from Mexico regularly return home to their families and are a potential source of TB transmission to their home areas.

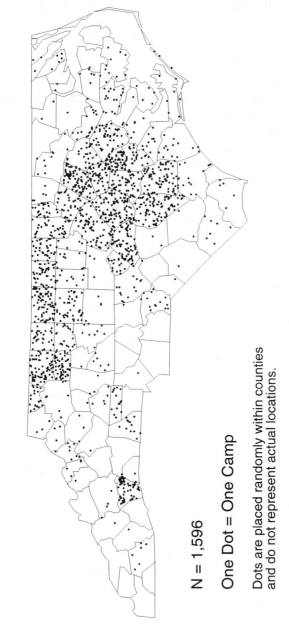

Figure 8-6   **NC Migrant Worker Camps, 1990**

N = 1,596

One Dot = One Camp

Dots are placed randomly within counties and do not represent actual locations.

Data Source: NC Department of Labor, 1991.
Produced by: North Carolina Rural Health Research Program, Cecil G. Sheps Center for Health Services Research, UNC - Chapel Hill.

Given our knowledge about changes in the disease and populations at risk for the disease, cartography can be used as a tool to
assess where TB health services should be concentrated. The
following series of maps (Figures 8-6 through 8-9) uses data from
the North Carolina Department of Labor and the North Carolina
Department of Environment, Health, and Natural Resources to
document the location of migrant workers in the state and those
counties with a high prevalence of TB. Figure 8-6 is a dot map,
which shows the general location of migrant housing camps in the
state.

Figures 8-7 through 8-9 display the TB rates per 100,000
population in each of the counties. The average rate of TB in North
Carolina in 1990 was 10 cases per 100,000, almost identical to the
national rate. In Figure 8-7, which shows rates for all races, there
is a band of counties in the eastern half of the state with prevailing
rates of tuberculosis much higher than the state and national
average. These counties "tend" in a northeast–southwest direction
from the Virginia to the South Carolina borders. Interstate 95, a
major north–south highway, runs through this area and, as a
transportation corridor, probably plays a part in the circulation of
tuberculosis in this part of the state. The counties in this area overlap
with the counties in Figure 8-6 containing the highest numbers of
migrant worker camps. Sampson (2,176), Nash (2,082), Johnston
(1,459), and Wilson (683) Counties have the largest populations of
migrant farm workers in this belt and are among the counties with
the highest rates of TB. Wilson County, with 30 cases of TB in
1990, had the highest rate of this group (45.4 cases per hundred
thousand). The band of counties along the northern border with
Virginia that contains a large number of migrant workers had only
average rates of TB. This difference might relate to the seasonality
of the crops in the two areas or the origin of the workers in the two
regions. The difference in rates invites further investigation.

Figure 8-8, which depicts the rate among whites in North
Carolina, shows no counties with rates much higher than the state
average except in six counties in the far eastern part of the state.

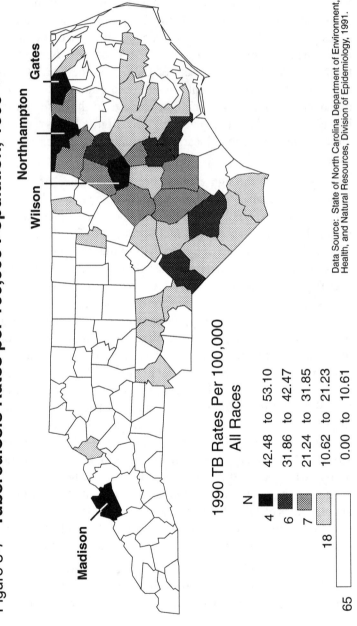

Figure 8-7 **Tuberculosis Rates per 100,000 Population, 1990**

1990 TB Rates Per 100,000
All Races

N		
4	42.48 to 53.10
6	31.86 to 42.47
7	21.24 to 31.85
18	10.62 to 21.23
65	0.00 to 10.61

Data Source: State of North Carolina Department of Environment,
Health, and Natural Resources, Division of Epidemiology, 1991.

Figure 8-9, which depicts the nonwhite TB rate, shows a clear pattern of high rates in the eastern part of the State. Almost a quarter of all counties in the state had TB rates above 30 per 100,000 among nonwhites.

Given limited outreach and treatment budgets, health departments faced with addressing the problem of the increasing prevalence of TB could use this simple cartographic means of reconnaissance to quickly pinpoint areas deserving closer examination in attempts to stop TB infection among migrant workers. For instance, if only two special TB programs could be funded in North Carolina, Wilson County and Sampson County would be likely targets— Wilson County, for the reasons mentioned above, and Sampson County because it had the largest number of farm workers in the State and had a TB rate of 31.7 per hundred thousand (more than three times the state and national average). On a more local scale, the location of migrant health centers, local hospitals, and places frequented by migrant farm workers could be identified on a map, targeting areas within these counties that would benefit most from more intensive TB control measures.

Concluding Comments

Understanding diffusion processes and mapping data on the distribution of epidemic cases as soon as those data become available can enable spatial modeling to predict the location of future occurrences, and can assist in the assessment of current health service needs at the local level. When available, mapping incidence data for tuberculosis, measles, or other contagious diseases on a demographic base map (see Chapter 3) would be even more useful in such assessments. At the county level, such maps can also be useful for communicating with local officials and the public, who sometimes think of disease as being present only in subgroups of the population in other places, rather than in their own community. At a state level, geographic models of the "gravity" or spatial autocorrelation families of models could be used to forecast future spatial distribution and service needs of high-impact disease such as AIDS where large prevention and education programs need to determine where to target their efforts.

Figure 8-8 **White Tuberculosis Rate per 100,000 Population, 1990**

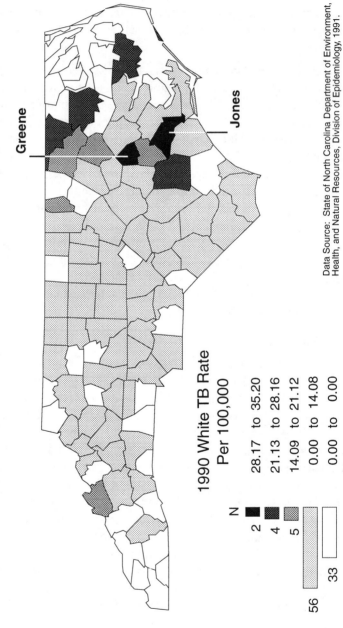

1990 White TB Rate
Per 100,000

N
2 ■ 28.17 to 35.20
4 ■ 21.13 to 28.16
5 ▨ 14.09 to 21.12
33 ▨ 0.00 to 14.08
56 □ 0.00 to 0.00

Greene

Jones

Data Source: State of North Carolina Department of Environment, Health, and Natural Resources, Division of Epidemiology, 1991.

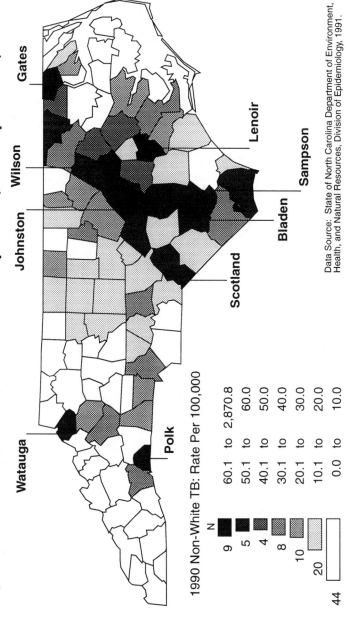

Figure 8-9 **Non-White Tuberculosis Rate per 100,000 Population, 1990**

1990 Non-White TB: Rate Per 100,000

9	60.1	to	2,870.8
5	50.1	to	60.0
4	40.1	to	50.0
8	30.1	to	40.0
10	20.1	to	30.0
20	10.1	to	20.0
44	0.0	to	10.0

Data Source: State of North Carolina Department of Environment, Health, and Natural Resources, Division of Epidemiology, 1991.

▷ P O I N T
▷ OF DEPARTURE

Adjustment of Tuberculosis Incidence Rates
Peter S. Millard

Tuberculosis (TB) is a communicable, bacterial disease spread almost exclusively person-to-person by airborne transmission. Most healthy people who are infected with TB do not develop symptoms but remain infected for years with inactive or *latent* disease. Only about ten percent of otherwise healthy people who have latent tuberculosis will eventually become ill with active TB. *Active TB disease* occurs when the infected person develops symptoms of TB (commonly consisting of cough, fever, night sweats, and weight loss). Most active disease results from reactivation of latent disease, months to many years after the initial infection.

Tuberculosis as a Public Health Problem

More than a century after the identification of the *Mycobacterium tuberculosis* organism, tuberculosis remains a serious public health problem. Throughout the world, ten million new cases are diagnosed and three million deaths occur from TB each year, accounting for six percent of all deaths (Sudre et al., 1992). Ten to fifteen million people in the United States have evidence of past infection with the TB bacillus and more than 125,000 persons receive preventive or therapeutic treatment for TB yearly (A strategic plan, 1989).

The US Tuberculosis Epidemic

After falling continuously by approximately six percent per year since national reporting began in 1953, TB incidence rates in the US leveled out in 1984 and began to increase in 1985. From 1985 to the end of 1991, there was an overall 18.4 percent increase in the number of active TB cases reported annually (Dooley et al., 1992).

Tuberculosis is a disease that occurs in the United States primarily among high-risk groups and in distinct geographic regions. Those at especially high risk for TB include HIV-infected persons, the homeless, immigrants from high-prevalence countries, intravenous drug users, prison inmates, and residents in long-term care facilities. TB is more common among men than women, and is twice as common among those over 65 years of age compared to those in the 15-44 age group (CDC, 1991b). Incidence rates among racial and ethnic minorities are four- to nine-fold higher than among non-Hispanic whites (CDC, 1991b).

Comparison of TB Incidence Rates

Epidemiologists commonly use several different methods to compare incidence rates between geographic areas (Hennekens & Buring, 1987). Comparisons can be made on the basis of crude incidence rates, stratum-specific rates, or standardized rates.

The *crude incidence rate* is calculated by dividing the number of new cases which occur over a given time period by the total population at risk for the disease. The crude incidence rate is vital for public health planning, but the use of crude rates to compare incidence rates across geographic areas is problematic. Variation in crude TB rates may occur solely due to differences in the age, race and gender distribution among populations, because the rate of tuberculosis varies significantly according to demographics. Thus, an area in which a large proportion of the population is elderly or nonwhite may have a high crude TB rate, but this rate may not be unexpected when one considers the makeup of the population.

Stratified analysis is one solution to this dilemma. Stratified analysis compares identical age-, race-, and gender-specific ("stratum-specific") categories in each geographic area. We would be comparing stratum-specific TB rates, for example, if we compared the rates among white males over the age of 65 years between two or more geographic areas. Unfortunately, stratified analysis results in a separate comparison for each category we choose, and there may be times when we prefer to summarize all the stratum-specific rates into a single figure.

Standardization, or *adjustment*, creates a single, summary rate for each geographic area. This is often more convenient than using multiple stratum-specific rates and may at the same time be free of the bias inherent in the use of crude rates. Standardization demands that the investigator first identify a *standard population* against which the adjusted rate can be directly compared. A standard population often comprises an area which includes the geographic areas to be compared. The US and world populations are frequently used as standard populations.

Direct standardization results in a single, adjusted rate for each geographic area. A directly-adjusted rate is a weighted average of stratum-specific rates. This rate is calculated in three steps:

1. Calculate a rate for each stratum by dividing the number of new cases in each stratum by the population in that stratum;

2. Calculate a weight for each stratum by dividing the population in each stratum by the population of the corresponding stratum in the standard population; and,

3. Multiply each stratum-specific rate by the corresponding stratum-specific weight and sum across all strata.

POINT OF DEPARTURE

The directly adjusted rate is equivalent to the crude rate which the geographic area of interest would have experienced if it had the same age, race, and gender distribution as the standard population.

Indirect standardization, on the other hand, can be used to calculate a *standardized incidence ratio,* which answers the question, "how does the adjusted rate compare to the crude rate in a standard population?" The standardized incidence ratio is calculated as follows:

1. Calculate the expected number of cases for each stratum by multiplying the population in each stratum by the rate for the corresponding stratum from the standard population;

2. Calculate the total expected cases for the geographic area by summing the expected number of cases over all strata; and,

3. Divide the total expected number of cases by the total observed number of cases in the geographic area.

A standardized incidence ratio of less than one indicates that the adjusted rate in the geographic area of interest is less than the rate in the standard population; a ratio of greater than one indicates the converse.

Direct standardization is easily interpreted, since it results in an actual rate which can be easily compared across geographic areas. However, indirect standardization allows a more precise comparison when the total number of cases in each stratum is low (fewer than ten cases for any age-, race-, or gender-specific stratum), since the directly adjusted rate may vary considerably due to random variation when there are few cases per stratum.

Both standardization procedures create a single summary number which allows for a straightforward comparison of rates between geographic areas. Stratum-specific rates, on the other hand, can be more revealing but are more difficult to interpret since they result in many simultaneous comparisons.

Indirect Standardization of TB Incidence Rates in North Carolina

We recently calculated standardized incidence ratios in order to compare TB rates among North Carolina counties for the period 1986-1990. We used indirect standardization since many age-, race-, and gender-specific strata had few TB cases. US national TB rates for the year 1988 served as the standard.

Compared to 1988 national rates, counties in western North Carolina have low TB rates. In contrast, 21 counties in eastern North Carolina have rates higher than the rest of the US (Figure 8-10).

We then stratified by age and simultaneously adjusted for race and gender. For those less than 25 years of age, rates are less than US rates for most counties in eastern North Carolina (Figure 8-11). For those aged 25 to 65 years, the pattern of high rates is evident; 13 counties have higher rates than the US (Figure 8-12). Eastern North Carolinians over 65 years of age have very high TB rates (Figure 8-13). Forty-four counties have higher rates than the rest of the nation and 24 counties have more than twice the national rate after adjustment for sex and race.

Conclusion

Standardization allows a valid comparison of TB incidence rates among North Carolina counties and shows a pattern of high rates in eastern North Carolina. Stratifying by age and standardizing by race and gender demonstrates that the increased incidence of TB in eastern North Carolina is primarily due to high rates in the elderly. Little active TB occurs in eastern North Carolina's youth, which suggests that little new transmission is occurring. High TB rates in the elderly of eastern North Carolina may be primarily due to reactivation of latent tuberculosis from past infection.

POINT OF DEPARTURE

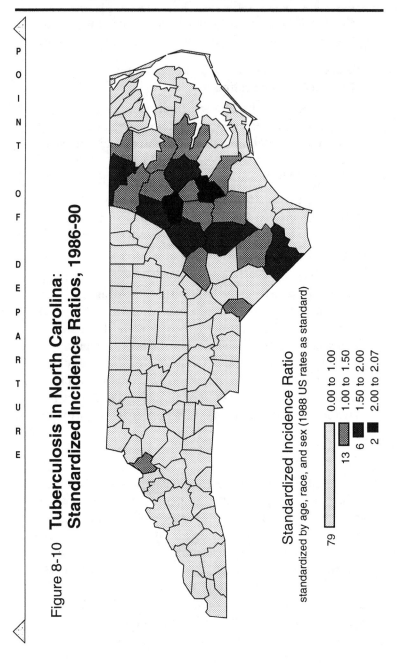

Figure 8-10 **Tuberculosis in North Carolina: Standardized Incidence Ratios, 1986-90**

Standardized Incidence Ratio

standardized by age, race, and sex (1988 US rates as standard)

79	0.00 to 1.00
13	1.00 to 1.50
6	1.50 to 2.00
2	2.00 to 2.07

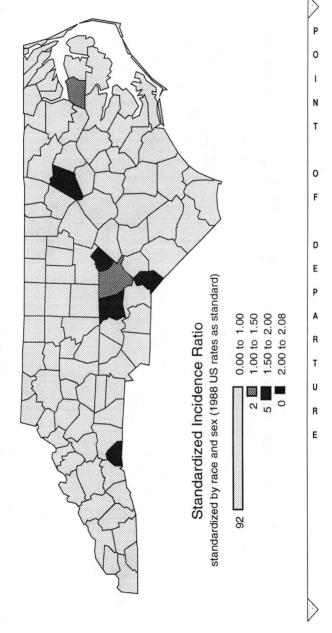

Figure 8-11 **Tuberculosis in North Carolina: Cases Aged Less than 25 Years Standardized Incidence Ratios, 1986-90**

Standardized Incidence Ratio

standardized by race and sex (1988 US rates as standard)

92   0.00 to 1.00

2   1.00 to 1.50

5   1.50 to 2.00

0   2.00 to 2.08

POINT OF DEPARTURE

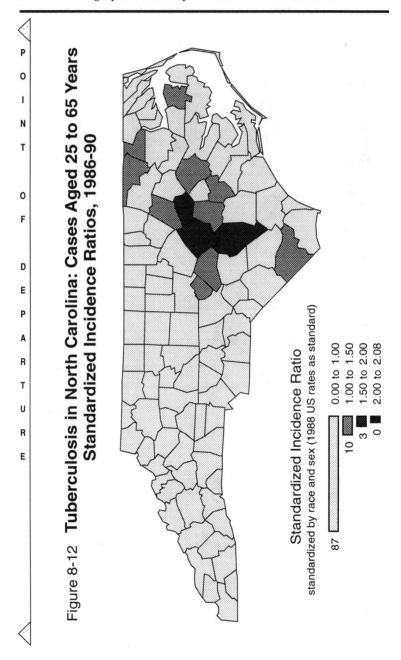

Figure 8-12   **Tuberculosis in North Carolina: Cases Aged 25 to 65 Years Standardized Incidence Ratios, 1986-90**

Standardized Incidence Ratio

standardized by race and sex (1988 US rates as standard)

0.00 to 1.00
1.00 to 1.50
1.50 to 2.00
2.00 to 2.08

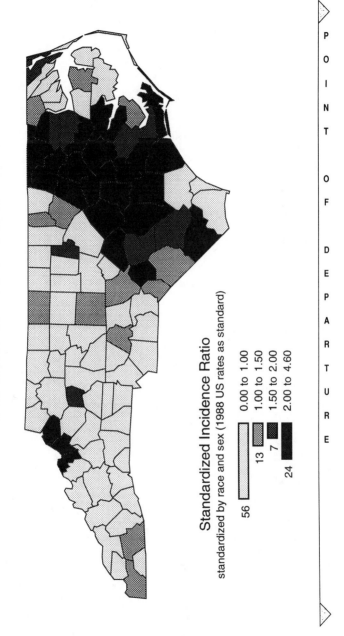

Figure 8-13   Tuberculosis in North Carolina: Cases Aged Greater than 65 Years
Standardized Incidence Ratios, 1986-90

Standardized Incidence Ratio
standardized by race and sex (1988 US rates as standard)

56   0.00 to 1.00
13   1.00 to 1.50
7   1.50 to 2.00
24   2.00 to 4.60

POINT OF DEPARTURE

Chapter 9

Evaluating Clusters
of Adverse Health Outcomes

Point of Departure:
State Cancer Control Program Map and Data Analyses

Introduction

The distribution of human characteristics is often described as random but also "normal," which is to say, the distribution of disease and disability can be predicted based on past observations. When the occurrence of disease or disability does not fit into an expected pattern, either by being unusually more common in one group of people, concentrated in one geographic area, or consolidated over a relatively short period of time, then we have reason to explore why these "clusters" or deviations from the normal pattern occur. This search for reasons is part of the regular work of the epidemiologist, who seeks to find factors in the environment, among the affected people, or in the nature of the disease that can explain this deviation from expectations.

The scientific basis of epidemiology depends on the predictable distribution of disease and disability in human populations (Doll, 1981). The principal activity in epidemiology is the careful examination of disease patterns—this is one reason that epidemiology is considered an observational science. Even when epidemiologists "test" hypotheses, they primarily do so through carefully selected observations called natural experiments and by comparing disease experiences between groups. Two examples of such exploratory analyses using descriptive data are subgroup analyses and cluster studies. Subgroup analyses are straightforward comparisons within a large data set, e.g., comparing brain cancer rates among children to those of other age groups. Cluster analyses seek to determine whether or not the observed number of cases of a disease is greater than would otherwise be expected. One also looks at the spatial pattern of cases within the defined geographic area, the time pattern for the occurrence of cases, and in some instances, the space-time pattern for any evidence that the distribution of cases is not random. This chapter will focus on the methods and application of cluster analysis, emphasizing spatial aspects. Examples are drawn from communities that illustrate specific approaches for cluster studies in rural places; these present special problems from a geographic perspective.

The Role of Public Health

The popular press increasingly describes potential disease cluster reports including birth defects, sudden infant death syndrome (SIDS), and, most commonly, cancer. Public health agencies are responsible for monitoring and responding to these reported events, usually through analysis of cancer incidence data at a variety of geographic scales. These studies can be used to provide surveillance information that may allay fears of the general public, prevent costly and unwarranted epidemiologic studies driven by political pressure, and target those reports warranting further investigation (Schneider et al., 1993). There are obvious public policy implications related to cluster reports as witnessed by Love Canal in the 1980's.

Most disease cluster reports are not, in fact, associated with increased occurrence, and even when increased disease rates are involved, currently accepted methods are often incapable of relating them to an environmental point source (Rothman, 1990; Neutra, 1990). Because of this inefficiency, evaluating disease cluster reports is a difficult and uncertain practice. However, researchers and health officials who choose to respond to cluster reports are greatly assisted by disease registries—in fact, some central registries came into being because of highly publicized cluster reports and the need for the population-based data that central registries can provide (Houk & Thacker, 1987; Aldrich et al., 1990).

Cluster studies are small-area investigations and usually involve very low numbers of cases (Thacker, 1989). These small numbers make the data analyses very subtle. A variety of specialized statistical methods have been developed for disease cluster analyses and computer software is available to assist with these analyses. These methods require the investigator to become familiarized with the analytic considerations and decision rules regarding the presence or absence of an identified cluster. Additionally, the investigator must subjectively decide which of the available tests are pertinent and should be applied to the potential clustering of the adverse health outcome being evaluated. The examples below depict those statistical tests selected in evaluating specific cancer "clusters" by a state health department.

The Notion of Clustering

An interesting development in health care research has been the use of a form of geographic regionalization to investigate the etiology of disease (Glaser, 1990; Ross & Davis, 1990). The use of these techniques to address regionalization issues is discussed briefly in Chapter 6. It is the former application, the investigation of disease etiology, which is the focus of this chapter. For these purposes, the specific location of each individual occurrence can be mapped to investigate the possibility of geographic clustering of occurrences. The underlying assumption is that a clustered (as opposed to random or uniform) pattern of distribution might sug-

Figure 9-1   **Clustered, Random, Uniform Distributions**

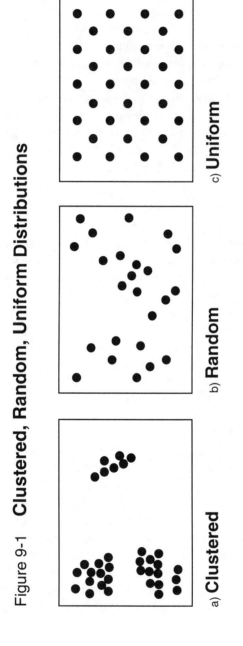

a) **Clustered**   b) **Random**   c) **Uniform**

Produced by: NC Rural Health Research Program, Cecil G. Sheps Center for Health Services Research, UNC - Chapel Hill.

gest a causal association (Figure 9-1). It might, however, merely suggest that the total population is clustered around that location. That potential problem can be addressed by using a cartogram with the unit size based on population rather than geographic area, as was depicted through the development of demographic base maps in Chapter 3.

Clustering involves a grouping of similar objects and has been widely applied, ranging from formal classification of plants and animals (dating back to Aristotle) to the detection of disease clusters (Hartigan, 1975). With respect to medicine, many varied adverse health outcomes have been analyzed using clustering analysis techniques. These include: SIDS (Grimson et al., 1981; Rodrigues et al., 1992), suicide (Gibbons & Clark, 1992), multiple sclerosis (Riise & Klauber, 1992), Hodgkin's disease (Ross & Davis, 1990), and cancer (Hatch et al., 1991; Glick, 1979; Ohno & Aoki, 1981). A special supplemental issue of the *American Journal of Epidemiology* (July, 1990) was compiled to report the proceedings from a national conference on the clustering of health events. Nevertheless, attention in the literature is most commonly focused on cancer clusters. For this reason, we have chosen to direct the remainder of this discussion to the evaluation of cancer clusters; however, these issues and techniques are germane to other adverse health events as well.

General Issues in
Evaluating Cancer Clusters

Three basic considerations must be kept in mind when evaluating cancer clusters. These are: 1) the identification process, 2) data availability and denominators, and 3) determination of the appropriate statistical approach for evaluation. These will be discussed below.

The identification process for cancer clusters should be a proactive versus reactive one. Ongoing surveillance on the part of a health department serves this function. A health department may gain access to evaluation software either by developing in-house capabilities (labor and capital) or through collaborative efforts with researchers at affiliated schools of public health and medicine. These analytic software packages together with informed scrutiny can be used to screen potential "hot spots." To standardize agency response, a protocol for responding to disease cluster reports should be developed. In North Carolina (Aldrich et al., 1990), the response protocol approach has enabled reports to be "closed," or found not to be excessive, after reviewing data for proximal populations (i.e., the surrounding county). It has been found that another large proportion of reports may be eliminated after a close review of the cases' clinical records (Heath, 1990) and removal of duplications in reporting associated with migration of cases or the same person being reported twice (e.g., children of divorced parents or maiden vs. married names for women; Schneider et al., 1993). The remaining reports are screened using statistical tests to distinguish the five to ten percent of all cluster reports received by an agency which will lead to new etiologic or disease control information.

Responding to disease cluster reports involves more than a search for disease etiology—after all, there are mental and social well being characteristics associated with "public health" (Bender et al., 1990). Providing cancer education is also part of being responsive to citizen concerns (Fiore et al., 1990). The identification process, in essence, serves a screening function, allowing scarce resources to be used to their greatest advantage. Further investigations can then be limited to those warranted by positive indications at this stage, while the fear of unwarranted reports may be dispelled.

One of the main difficulties encountered in research using medical geography is the availability of consistent and reliable data—especially data sources that cross geopolitical borders. For public health officers, state cancer registries are an important source of data. Many areas do not have registries; some that do have not collected data that are particularly meaningful for the analysis of cancer. Difficulties associated with the reliability and comparability of data along both spatial and temporal gradients need to be considered. For example, variations across cancer registries in coding the site of the lesion as well as the stage of diagnosis for certain cancers, which may require sophisticated technology and/or professional specialization, should be understood when comparing data from separate reporting sources. Schneider et al. (1993) found that cancer clusters could not be detected consistently across scales and caution researchers to select a scale that is most consistent with the etiology of the cancer being evaluated. Finally, the small numbers associated with a relatively rare event such as cancer mean that there will be statistical instability in the rates used for evaluative purposes—the denominator problem. Verhasselt (1977) presents an interesting overview of these concerns and Shafer (1980) discusses relevant considerations for mapping cancer.

To the extent that a cluster has been identified and appropriate data are available, the investigator is then charged with determining the appropriate approach to use in the evaluation. There are quite a few different approaches available. Table 9-1 summarizes those considered in evaluating the case examples in this chapter. References to these are provided for in-depth clarification and interested readers are referred to an issue of *Morbidity and Mortality Weekly Report* on this topic that presents a very thorough and concise discussion of each individual method (CDC, 1990). These approaches vary, however, in their ability to detect clusters with differential characteristics. We have found that it is a good strategy to use more than one statistical approach or method to assess evidence of unusual disease aggregation. Analytic statistical methods can be classified into the distinct categories of case data, cell data, and surveillance. Results from these should generally agree and this consistency between findings acts to reinforce results that may be of borderline statistical significance ($p < 0.06$). With multiple statistical methods being used, agreement by three or more methods (our criteria) may be regarded as remarkable. If five or more methods agree, this is cause for overwhelming attention to the clustering event.

The evaluation of clusters requires detailed information and sometimes exhaustive background research. Geographic informa-

Table 9-1

Statistical Tests for Assessing Clusters
of Adverse Health Events

Temporal Clustering

Scan Test   The maximum number of cases observed over a given time segment is determined by scanning all time segments within an overall time period, which results in overlapping time periods. P-values are used to test for statistical significance.

Reference: Naus JI. 1982. Approximations for Distributions of Scan Statistics. *Journal of American Statistical Association* 77:177-83.

Chen Test   This test identifies evidence of temporal clustering on the basis of the shortening of the interval between case occurrences. Cases are chronologically ordered and the expected number of cases is computed for comparison. P-values are used to test for the statistical significance of the observed-to-expected ratios.

Reference: Chen R. 1986. Revised Values for the Parameters of the Sets Technique for Monitoring the Incidence Rate of a Rare Disease. *Methods of Information in Medicine* 25:47-49.

Poisson Test   This test seeks to evaluate rates over time. For each specified time interval, the observed and expected rates are compared using a Poisson solution for acceptably small rates. Again, p-values are used to assess statistical significance.

Reference: Hill GB, Spicer CC, Weatherall JAC. 1968. The Computer Surveillance for Congenital Malformations. *British Medical Bulletin* 24:215-218.

Texas Test   This test seeks to evaluate the temporal pattern for rare health events over a specified time period. For each interval, the observed and expected rates are compared using a Poisson solution for acceptably small rates and a modified binomial for larger rates. P-values are used to assess statistical significance.

Reference: Hardy RJ, Schroeder GD, Cooper SP, Buffler PA, et al. 1990. A Surveillance System for Assessing Health Effects from Hazardous Exposures. *American Journal of Epidemiology* 132:S-S.

Spatial Clustering

Grimson Test   This test was developed as a test of spatial clustering for use in identifying clusters of geographic areas designated as "high risk." The test statistic is the number of pairs of high-risk areas that are adjacent to each other. Monte Carlo simulation is used to generate p-values to test the statistical significance of the test statistic.

Reference: Grimson RC, Wang KC, and Johnson PWC. 1981. Searching for Hierarchical Clusters of Disease, Spatial Patterns of Sudden Infant Death Syndrome. *Social Science and Medicine* 15:287-93.

Ohno Test   This test uses rates for geographic areas rather than individual, case-specific data. The similarity of rates between adjacent areas is compared. The test statistic is the number of concordant pairs. The observed versus the expected number of concordant pairs is compared using a chi-square test to assess statistical significance.

Reference: Ohno Y and Aoki K. 1981. Cancer Deaths by City and County in Japan 1969-1971: A Test of Significance for Geographic Clusters of Disease. *Social Science and Medicine* 15D:251-258.

Spatial & Temporal Clustering

Knox Test   This is a 2 x 2 contingency table test that dichotomizes the spatial and temporal aspects of the potential cluster. The contingency table is formed by classifying pairs of cases based upon their relative proximity in both space and time. The test statistic, X, is the observed number of pairs close in both space and time, which approximates the Poisson distribution.

Reference: Knox EG. 1964. The Detection of Space-Time Interactions. *Applied Statistics* 13:25-29.

Barton Test   This test involves clustering (with respect to time) pairs of cases separated in time by some predetermined maximum time segment (e.g., less than 2 years). The test statistic, Q, is the ratio of the average squared geographic distance between all pairs of cases. Calculation of the distribution of statistical significance testing can be problematic; using a randomization test to determine the distribution, a beta approximation when the number of cases is small, and a normal distribution when the number of cases is large have all been suggested.

Reference: Barton DE, David FN, Merrington M. 1965. A Criterion for Testing Contagion in Time and Space. *Annals of Human Genetics* 29:97-101.

REMSA   This test is a simple probability evaluation. For each of the characteristics under consideration (e.g., space, time, demographic, social), a cluster cell is constructed with its own associated probability. Statistical significance for generated probabilities is assessed using p-values.

Reference: Aldrich TE, Wilson CC, Easterly CE. 1985. Population Surveillance for Rare Health Events. Proceedings, 1985 Public Health Conference on Records and Statistics, DHHS Publication No. 86-1214, pp. 215-220.

tion systems (GIS) have made this task somewhat easier from a measurement perspective. These systems link databases of population demographics to some geographic feature (e.g., address information, latitude/longitude coordinates, Census tracts, industrial locations, hazardous waste sites) and permit spatial analysis through overlay maps. In this way, a variety of information can be overlayed, possibly identifying problematic areas for further investigation. GIS also provides analysts with the ability to examine areas that cross geopolitical borders. Several examples of the power of these analyses are provided below and a thoughtful discussion of GIS is provided in the Point of Departure on that topic, which is included in Chapter 6.

Applications

We would like to illustrate cancer cluster analysis by providing three examples of clusters that were evaluated through the North Carolina Cancer Registry using the CLUSTER® software (see the Technical Notes for acquisition information) along with basic investigative epidemiologic techniques. Statistical significance is measured using the p-value which is discussed in most introductory statistics texts; the conventional 0.05 level of significance is used in these analyses. The examples will serve to highlight the points made in our previous discussion. Each of these examples begins with a brief overview of the case, is followed by a discussion of the cluster analysis and concludes with a summary of results.

Pancreatic Cancer in Ashe and Alleghany Counties

Initially, a report of a cancer cluster led to an inspection of cancer rates for Ashe County, North Carolina. That particular report was not borne out by further study, yet continued surveillance was indicated (Aldrich et al., 1991). During the course of the surveillance, so-called "sentinel" cancers were inspected (Aldrich et al., 1989). Sentinel cancers are rare cancers suspected of having a potential association with environmental exposures (Rothwell et al., 1991). Elevated rates of pancreatic cancer were observed for both Ashe and Alleghany counties and the evaluation for evidence of county-level aggregates was statistically significant (other elevated county rates were not seen in contiguous counties). At about this same time, a local physician also noted the rise in diagnoses of pancreatic cancers in Alleghany County and called the pattern to the attention of the Cancer Surveillance Unit (CSU). These stimuli prompted this special study. Pancreatic cancer is quite rare—its incidence in the United States is only 9.1 per 100,000 persons per year; rates have been observed to be slightly higher for males and for blacks.

All pancreatic cancer cases occurring among residents of Ashe and Alleghany Counties during the period 1980-1989 were identified. The majority of the cases were deceased and were identified through vital records; other cases were located via physician offices and reporting to the North Carolina Central Cancer Registry. Information was collected for general descriptive characteristics from these data sources (e.g., age, race, sex, place of residence at the time of diagnosis). For each case, residence at the time of diagnosis/ death was assigned geographic coordinates using maps from the US Geological Survey (Figure 9-2). Staff members of the Ashe and Alleghany County Health Departments helped State investigators in determining meaningful geographic boundaries and worked diligently canvassing the community to verify addresses (many were rural routes) and to establish residency duration (cases living in either county for fewer than ten years were excluded from the analysis). Additionally, environmental health staff collected information on pesticide use practices for their respective counties for the 1970 to 1985 period.

Cluster Analysis: Fifty-one incident pancreatic cancer cases were identified for the decade of the 1980's among residents of these two counties (combined 1990 population 31,401) with three case exclusions due to short residency. Simple comparisons of the crude rates and space–time cluster analyses were used to search for evidence of nonrandom distribution of the cases or clusters of cases within the larger, two-county area. The overall annual crude incidence rate was 16.24 (the age-adjusted rate was 11.3).

Figure 9-2   **Residence-at-Diagnosis, Pancreatic Cancer Cases Studied Using Arbitrary Boundaries within Ashe and Alleghany Counties**

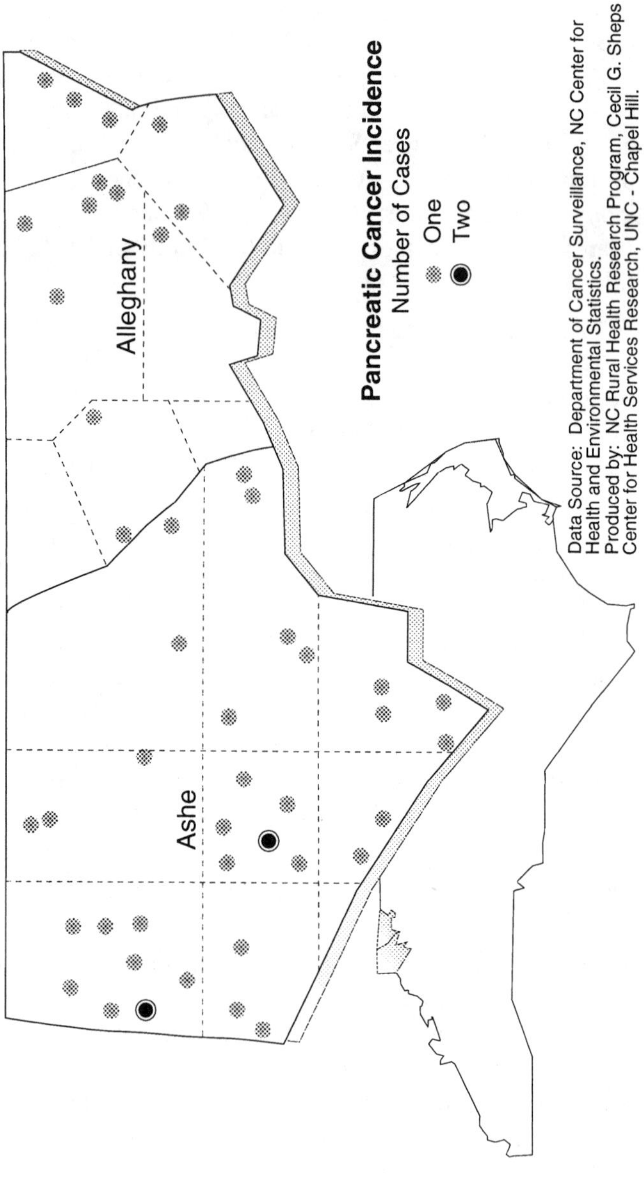

Analyses for evidence of space–time clustering were conducted using five statistical methods selected from the array of those available in the software program: Knox, Barton, Scan, Texas, and Poisson. These particular tests were selected based on their sensitivity to pertinent aspects of the potential cluster being scrutinized. The tests are identified by their major proponents or convention among investigators familiar with these studies (refer to Table 9-1 for more information on individual test properties). Results from each of these are summarized below:

Knox: This test for space–time clustering was based on five spatial units (a convention used for most previous cluster analyses in North Carolina). Two years were selected as a time period for designating "closeness." These delimiters found 34 observed case pairs "close" in space and time, where 29 would have been expected by chance alone (p > 0.18).

Barton: This test examines the spatial distribution of cases by their temporal distribution. With this test, no evidence of clustering was found.

Scan: This test looks for evidence of increased clustering in time. A two-year window was used to scan, i.e., nine windows in all. For 48 cases, 9.6 cases might have been expected in any one window; 17 cases (1987-88) were observed (p > 0.21).

Texas: This test is especially useful for studying small area rates over time. For 1987, the test showed statistical significance, but as 1988 and all other years were included, this single year increase is regarded as a random "swing."

Poisson: This test's result agreed with the Texas findings. An attempt to evaluate a run of individual time periods using the Negative Binomial option was also not statistically significant.

In addition, simple comparisons of the crude rates using convenient, arbitrary geographic regions of the two counties were used to locate higher occurrence areas. These are depicted in Figure 9-2. Visual inspection suggested elevated occurrence in several of the regions. Some of these areas were adjacent. Reports from the county agricultural extension agents in Ashe County indicated the highest use of those pesticides of interest in two of the regions of high occurrence as well as generally higher use for all reported pesticides during the time period 1970-85.

Several cases, which were located near each other, were selected among those occurring during the 1987 and 1988 high occurrence interval. Survivors of these seven cases were interviewed; interview questions focused on presence of the risk factors for cancer reported in the published literature. The interview results failed to reveal any meaningful associations whatsoever. All women were housewives, the men did not work in the same industries or locations, and three of the women had diabetes or a history of it in their families. None of the cases shared common water supplies or reported remarkable pesticide exposures. None of the cases reported common social contacts (e.g., church attendance); and no unusual proportion reported high-risk lifestyles (e.g., alcohol, coffee, smoking).

Results: The agency concluded that there was no apparent explanation for these increased rates of pancreatic cancer. The possibility of age-specific effects leading to higher rates than those calculated with age adjustment may exist due to several cases being quite old and an increasing pattern of retired persons migrating into the area. The one very young case in Alleghany County (age 40 years) would also have an impact on the age-adjusted rates. However, after the removal of recent residents, some regions of higher occurrence persisted, affirming that the potential for increased risk was present. Surveillance for any change in rates will continue for these counties over the next five years although the rates for the counties have already been observed to be decreasing. Five cases occurred in 1990, two in Alleghany (both males) and three in Ashe (two men and one woman). Their occurrence had no impact on the regional, crude rates.

Cluster Report—Wilkes County, North Carolina

This evaluation was begun in May, 1991, as the culmination of efforts by a local community organization. Data collection was completed in August, with a second submission of data received in December of that year. Efforts were made to verify the case data collected; the data were then analyzed for spatial, temporal, and space–time patterns. The incidence of cancer in this community of about 700 persons was significantly higher than the expected (national) rates.

In all, 89 people were identified as cancer cases through the community survey. Twenty-two of these were excluded due to: diagnoses before the study period (1980-89), common skin cancers, and pre-malignant conditions (e.g., cervical dysplasia). Three additional cancer cases were identified via hospital record reviews, death certificate searches, and review of the 1987-89 partial cancer registry data. For 1990, five new cancer cases were identified from this area; the sites of these cancers are listed in Table 9-2. With partial data in 1991, four cases were identified.

Thus, 70 cases were considered for this analysis. For these cases, 34 were males, 36 females; all were white. The age distribution of the cases was skewed toward older ages (only one pediatric cancer was found); this is consistent with the age distribution for cancer incidence and for the study community. The majority of the cancers identified were of expected sites (e.g., lung, breast, colon). Using national data, 24 cases would have been expected for the estimated 700 residents (based on the survey) over this ten-year period. Using population distribution data from the 1990 Census for the Census tract that encompasses these 13 tax parcels, age-adjusted rates were calculated (adjusted to the US 1970 Census population so that direct comparison with national data is possible). The three-fold overall increase is noteworthy and is statistically significant ($p < 0.05$). However, the certainty of the actual population represented may be questioned (because of in- and out-migration of residents). Simple standardized incidence ratios (SIR) are shown in Table 9-2 as well.

Cluster Analysis: Evidence of increased cancer mortality for several cancers in Wilkes County during the decade of the 1980's had already been identified. These mortality increases were based

Table 9-2
Cancer Cases for the Wilkes County Cluster Area (1980-89)

Site of Cancer	1980	1981	1982	1983	1984	1985	1986	1987	1988	1989	Total	SIR*
Lung	1	1		1		2	4	2		1	12	**2.6**
Colon	1			2		2	1	1		1	9	**3.4**
Breast	2	2		1	1				2	1	10	1.3
Prostate			1					2	1	1	5	
Leukemia	1					2	1				4	**7.2**
Lymphoma	1						1	1	1	1	5	**4.4**
Stomach						2					2	
Liver								1			1	
Pancreas								1		1	2	4.3
Melanoma			1	1		2					4	
Brain				1	1	1	1		1		5	**11.8**
Kidney			1	1							2	
All Other	1	2					4	1	1		9	
Total	7	5	3	7	3	11	12	10	6	6	70	**3.0**

1990 cases: one colon, two lung, one leukemia and one lymphoma.
* Selected sites only, age-adjusted to the 1970 US Census and compared with national data.
p < 0.05 are in **bold**.

on race- and sex-specific, age-adjusted mortality rates (uniformly adjusted to the 1970 US Census) and the observed mortality increases were relatively consistent throughout the decade. For this analysis, 20 cancers that may have had environmental associations were examined (even though some sites did not represent increased numbers of cases, e.g., liver, testes, and kidney). The leukemia, lymphoma, and brain cancer data were also analyzed separately as these rates were most increased among the selected "environmental" cancers. Six cluster tests were chosen for this analysis. Again, interested readers are referred to Table 9-1 for specific references and properties associated with the tests. Results from those tests utilized in this particular investigation are summarized below:

Knox: This test for space–time clustering was based on 10 spatial units (Figure 9-3). Two years were used as a time period for designating "closeness." These delimiters found 12 observed case pairs "close" in space and time, where 15 would have been expected by chance alone ($p > 0.80$). Neither brain cancer, leukemia nor lymphoma showed evidence of disease clustering ($p > 0.57$) with one observed pair and two expected for lymphoma and brain and six observed and expected for leukemia.

Barton: This test seeks explanation of a spatial distribution by the temporal distribution (again for mixed sites of cancer). The result detected the 1985-87 cases. It failed to detect clustering for lymphoma or brain cancer cases (both have no years with multiple cases). Leukemia was increased again because of the 1985-86 years.

Scan: This test looks for evidence of disease clustering in time. A three-year window was used to scan, i.e., eight windows in all. For all 20 cases, six cases might have been expected in any one window; 11 cases were observed (1985-87; $p < 0.22$). Lymphoma and brain cancer data were too widely spaced in time for use with this method. With leukemia and lymphoma together, five cases were observed, 2.7 expected ($p < 0.69$).

REMSA: This technique, using all 20 cases, did not show an unusual aggregation despite a leukemia and two lymphomas in one

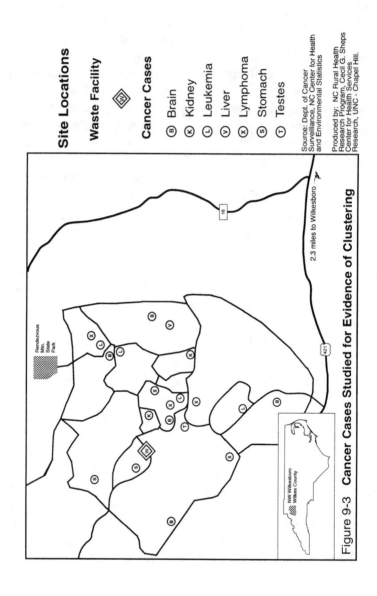

Site Locations

Waste Facility

⊛ W

Cancer Cases

ⓑ Brain
ⓚ Kidney
ⓛ Leukemia
ⓥ Liver
ⓧ Lymphoma
ⓢ Stomach
ⓣ Testes

Source: Dept. of Cancer
Surveillance, NC Center for Health
and Environmental Statistics

Produced by: NC Rural Health
Research Program, Cecil G. Sheps
Center for Health Services
Research, UNC - Chapel Hill.

Figure 9-3   **Cancer Cases Studied for Evidence of Clustering**

tax district (p < 0.274). However, the cases were dissimilar in all other characteristics (age, sex, cell type). With brain cancer, there was no evidence of an unusual pattern in space or time. The leukemia cases were among older persons; also the cell types were not consistent.

Texas: This test is especially useful for studying small area rates over time. All 70 of the cancer cases were used with this analysis. For 1985 through 1987, the test showed statistical significance (p < 0.001); this is likely the pattern of increased occurrence that the community recognized.

Poisson: This result agreed with the Texas findings (significantly increased in 1985-87). An attempt to evaluate a run of individual time periods using the Negative Binomial option was also significant for 1985-87 with p < 0.05.

Results: The period 1985-87 represented unusual frequencies of cancer cases. However, lung cancer was the only anatomic site where a large increase was seen for these years. Also, there are significantly increased rates for colon, leukemia, lymphoma, and brain cancer. For these cancers, no space or time grouping was found.

The elevated colon and lung cancer rates are interesting, yet the strong association of these cancers with lifestyle factors (e.g., smoking and diet) call for less attention in this evaluation. The two pancreatic cancers occurring in this community may be related to a regional pattern of increased occurrence in two contiguous counties to the north of Wilkes County. This same "regional" effect may be true for both brain cancer (among counties to the south) and lymphoma (counties to the west). Because of the already identified "regional" concerns for brain and pancreatic cancer, cases from this community will be included with studies on a larger geographic scale.

The overall higher occurrence of cancer in this community is clear. Similarly, the increases for leukemia, lymphoma, and brain cancer raise concerns for an environmental risk. As monitoring around the waste disposal site has not shown any evidence of hazardous materials escaping into the environment, there was no basis for further study of the cancer risk within the community based upon its location near the site. This evaluation was closed with the direction that further epidemiologic surveillance be conducted in light of the overall elevated numbers of cancers in this community.

Three-County Brain Cancer Study

A potential cluster of brain cancer cases in Rowan County was received from a local physician. Further evaluation of the cluster did not support a generalized increase for brain cancer, yet there were some peculiar geographic and temporal patterns (Aldrich et al., 1991). A follow-up study was organized to use GIS techniques to further evaluate these patterns. The study area was expanded to encompass the two neighboring counties (Davie County, which had elevated brain cancer rates, and Davidson County).

The GIS database used for this study contains information on licensed industry dischargers, national priority list (Superfund) hazardous waste sites, high-voltage electrical power lines (more than 100kV), and provocative rural exposure (commercial chicken farms—linked with brain cancer from earlier brain cancer cluster reports). The cases included in this study are all incident brain cancers from 1980-89 and include 130 malignant brain cancers and 159 controls (septicemia deaths for the same time period). Staff members of the CSU mapped the residences of 121 (93%) of the cases and 150 (94%) of the controls; missing addresses were either post office boxes or simply could not be located.

The community of Cooleemee, North Carolina, which is located in both Davie and Rowan counties, was of particular interest for this study because of an earlier cluster report. Figure 9-4 shows the three-county study area with the symmetric geographic areas used in the preliminary analysis. This diagram exemplifies the type of geographic referencing that is possible with GIS, in this instance looking at brain cancer risk in Cooleemee, a community in the south

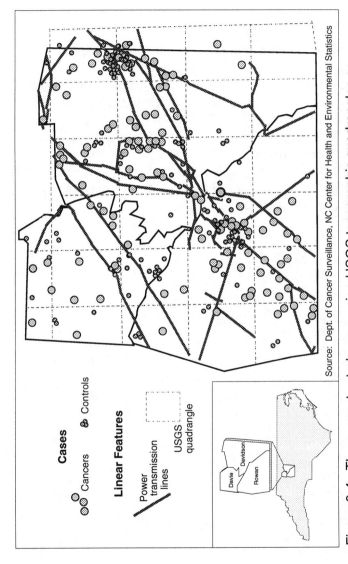

Figure 9-4 Three-county study area using USGS topographic quadrangles as internal boundaries. Clusters analyzed by proximity to power transmission lines.

center of Davie County that spans the county line. Without the level of precision available through GIS, investigations are confined to areas lying within geopolitical borders as cross-border studies are often severely limited in their ability to analyze data at this scale of analysis.

Cluster Analysis and Results: For this analysis, the 1986-87 national brain cancer incidence rate (6.2 per 100,000 persons) was used to arrive at an expected number of brain cancer cases for comparison to the observed cases. (See Chapter 6, *Health Professions Distributions*, for a discussion of the observed-to-expected ratio calculation.) During the decade of 1980-1989, 130 cases of brain cancer were observed for the three-county study area (SIR = 130/158.4 = 0.82, p < 0.50). None of the county-specific risk estimates are statistically significant and only Davie County's rate was increased (Table 9-3).

Table 9-3
Annual Brain Cancer Cases By Year
(Three-County Region, 1980-89)

Year	Rowan County	Davie County	Davidson County	
1980	4	4	3	
1981	4	3	8	
1982	0	3	3	
1983	5	1	10	
1984	2	1	6	
1985	7	1	7	
1986	7	1	6	
1987	6	5	7	
1988	6	2	9	
1989	5	0	4	
				TOTAL
TOTAL	46	21	63	130
Expected Cases	71.9	15.7	70.8	158.4
Standardized Incidence Ratios	0.64	1.34	0.89	0.82

The study evaluated residential proximity to the various environmental point sources available in the database. A residential proximity threshold of 500 feet was used in defining "close." Elevated risk assessments (i.e., calculated odds ratios) were not found for industrial dischargers, electrical substations, Superfund sites, or chicken farms. Only residential proximity to electric power lines showed evidence of an increased risk, and the risk estimates increased for closer distances (maximum at 125 feet) but were unreliable due to the small numbers. These results indicate the substantial capability of a GIS for geographic proximity studies—even to distances of hundreds of feet—which previously were not possible.

Another tactic involves studies of small geographic areas below the county level and along or across county lines. An analysis of cancer rates around Cooleemee Township, which is located in the North Carolina piedmont, is an example of such a strategic area that spans county lines. Earlier studies of possibly increased cancer rates in Cooleemee had been hampered by the difficulty of studying disease rates for portions of a county. GIS techniques overcome these difficulties. Each of the small geographic areas represents a specific portion of the population for the study area; this is represented by the distribution of comparison addresses (Table 9-4). A simple proportional ratio measure (proportion of case addresses divided by proportion of comparison addresses) was used to evaluate evidence of increased brain cancer occurrence within these small geographic areas.

The proportional analysis from these 24 geographic areas was quite interesting. Cooleemee was not shown to have evidence of an elevated brain cancer risk. Using the guidelines of the current cluster protocol, only Midway, Lexington East, Rowan Mills, and China Grove would be considered remarkable observations (none of the increases found for the individual small geographic areas are statistically significant). However, attention must be given to the proximity of pairs of these areas (see Figure 9-4). The increased brain cancer occurrence for the combined area of Rowan Mills and

Table 9-4

Brain Cancer Risk Estimates, 1980-89

Risk Estimates (Proportional Address Ratios) by County Small
Divisions for Three-County Study of Brain Cancer, 1980-89
(Septicemia Deaths as Comparison Addresses)

Division	Cases	Controls	Ratio	
Calahan	1	3	n/a	
Mocksville	4	7	0.71	
Advance	4	3	1.67	
Welcome	8	4	2.50	
Midway	4	1	5.00	*
High Point	8	13	0.77	
Cool Spring	1	1	n/a	
Colleemee	5	12	0.52	
Churchland	1	1	n/a	
Lexington W	14	12	1.46	
Lexington E	7	1	8.74	*
Fair Grove	7	24	0.36	
Cleveland	1	3	n/a	
Rowan Mills	8	2	5.00	*
Salisbury	16	39	0.51	
Southmont	5	0	n/a	#
Grist Mtn	1	1	n/a	
Denton	3	0	n/a	#
Enochville	5	3	2.08	
China Grove	11	2	6.88	**
Rockwell	2	4	0.62	
Gold Hill	0	1	n/a	
High Rock	0	0	0.00	
Handy	0	0	0.00	
Total	116	145		
Edge Areas	5	5	not included	

* Small geographic areas indicating increased brain cancer occurrence.
  All are not statistically significant ($p > 0.05$).
\# Not calculated with zero controls.
** Identified as having higher rates from the earlier cluster study.

China Grove is statistically significant. This evidence of increased occurrence reinforces the preliminary results from an earlier brain cancer cluster report that had been received for Rowan County. For the Welcome, Midway, and Lexington East areas, 3 contiguous areas with proportional ratios greater than 1.0, the combined proportional ratio is not statistically significant.

These findings of proportional increases in contiguous areas are curious. On detailed inspection of the cases, no further consistency was identified to clarify risk factors. The cases from these contiguous areas were of various ages and both races and sexes. Additionally, they were not spatially grouped within the small geographic areas, nor did they cluster along shared area borders. The cases were not particularly close to any of the other study point sources (industrial sites, poultry farms, substations, etc.). Nonetheless, it was exciting to be able to identify small geographic areas, below the county level, for performing such detailed case studies (Armenian, 1991).

The ease and rapidity of this special study of a small geographic area was encouraging. Future analyses using these GIS techniques (without the costly field work for data collection) will greatly extend cancer surveillance capabilities for the State. Geographic files from the 1990 Census are available and will further augment this resource.

The evaluation of disease cluster reports would seem to be a permanent fixture in public health practice, as is the public's concern with environmental protection (Fiore et al., 1990). The Cancer Surveillance Section of the Division of Statistics and Information Services in the North Carolina Department of Environment, Health, and Natural Resources receives, on average, three reports per month that must be addressed. Public health agencies are in need of technology to promote general welfare in the face of the public's apparent wish to have both a highly industrialized society and a safe environment (Ruckelshous, 1984). Tests to detect disease clustering, while not designed to estimate disease risk, may be used to alert agencies to potential need and to assist with decision making (Glasser, 1985). They may also be used to target public education programs for identified areas of potential need.

Disease surveillance is an established part of public health practice (Thacker & Berkelman, 1988). Increasingly, there are available population-based resources for public health surveillance since the majority of states now have cancer registries. With the persistent problem of incoming disease cluster reports to consider, a particular surveillance strategy is recommended that could provide a proactive approach to disease clustering. This is the systematic monitoring of disease occurrence patterns expressly used to detect unusual case aggregations before they present themselves as a cluster "report." For this purpose, we recommend the selection of strategic, rare health events as sentinels of potential exposure to hazardous substances in the environment (Rothwell et al., 1991). Rare health events may serve public health surveillance purposes particularly well because of the small numbers of events needed for decision making and because of their greater plausibility for having environmental etiologies.

Active responses to reports of small area disease aggregates (clusters) may prove a useful means for encouraging a dialogue between concerned citizens and agency representatives, as suggested by Fiore et al. (1990). However, such systematic processes must be carefully organized around a consistent protocol and should be guided by statistical methods applied as a screen for selecting promising reports for further studies. The discipline of epidemiology should move forward with developing new cluster identification methods for use with population-based disease surveillance of environmental health concerns.

P O I N T
OF DEPARTURE

P
O
I
N
T

O
F

D
E
P
A
R
T
U
R
E

State Cancer Control Map and Data Program: Analysis of Unusual Mortality Patterns
Forrest Pommerenke

Public health officials need to respond quickly to reports of unusual cancer clusters or alarming cancer mortality trends. A personal computer program has been developed that provides detailed state and county cancer mortality statistics and maps that can help in the analysis of unusual cancer patterns at state and county levels. It can also serve as a monitoring tool for public health officials in targeting areas of underservice for oncology services as well as potential areas for education and early detection interventions.

Overview of the Computer Program

The *State Cancer Control Map and Data Program* (SCCMDP)[1] produces state-level maps and printed data tables according to the user's choice of six parameters listed on a simple menu on the computer screen. These basic parameters include: 1) state and/or county, 2) type of cancer, 3) gender and race, 4) age range of population of interest, and 5) time period between 1953 and 1987. Once the parameters have been selected, the program calculates the rates and creates maps showing the relative mortality rates for each county within the state.

[1]The SCCMDP was developed by Aurest Inc., of Clifton, Virginia and the Early Detection Branch, Division of Cancer Prevention and Control, National Cancer Institute, Bethesda, Maryland. The Centers for Disease Control and the American Cancer Society also participated in the design and support of the program.

Choroplethic maps produced by the program give a graphic display of the data. The maps created by SCCMDP use different colors to illustrate cancer rates at the county level. Counties with rates that are significantly higher than national averages are red, those with significantly high rates that are at least 33 percent above the national average are deep red, those with average rates are yellow, and those with low rates are green. The system is based on color representations and output requires a color system.

All of the data in the program can also be printed as tables. The state tables, for example, list all of the state's counties in rank order by: 1) age-adjusted rates (highest rate first), 2) number of deaths (largest number of deaths listed first), or 3) alphabetical order (see Tables 9-5 and 9-6 for examples of output). The data can be further summarized in tables to show the statistics from within individual counties. These county-specific tables list the number of deaths and the age-specific rates for each age group (from 0-4 through 85 and older) for each time period between 1953-1957 to 1983-1987 (see Table 9-7).

Application of Mortality Maps and Data

The SCCMDP is intended to enable local public health planners to analyze their own cancer mortality patterns so that they can use cartography in targeting their efforts toward the cancers and populations that cause the greatest mortality. For example, using data from the program, a user could determine the change over the past twenty years in lung cancer mortality in a particular county. These data might be helpful in passing local ordinances to restrict smoking in public places. Local statistics could also be used in educational efforts to increase public awareness about the importance of early cancer detection.

The computer program can also be utilized to investigate unusual cancer mortality patterns and to respond to public anxiety regarding possible cancer clusters. These concerns, in the absence of accurate information, may lead to unnecessary public worry and unsubstantiated allegations that may, in fact, be unwarranted. The following examples illustrate how the program has been able to provide quick and reliable information regarding reports of unusual cancer mortality patterns.

Clarifying rates. A report of an 80 percent increase in breast cancer mortality over a five-year period in a New England state provided an early opportunity to use the SCCMDP. The program allowed a local public health official to perform a mortality analysis and to respond in time to prevent needless public anxiety. The official found that the misleading report relied on statistics that were calculated on the basis of only a few deaths each year. This common statistical error results in rates that can vary widely and can be interpreted (or misinterpreted) to be increasing or decreasing depending upon which years were compared. Without the SCCMDP, this particular public health official might not have been able to respond promptly. Delay, in this case, could have provided silent support for a poorly corroborated report.

Refuting associations. A recent report linked fluoride to bone cancer in laboratory animals. This report was enough to commission several high-level investigations looking for similar associations in human populations with high levels of fluoride in their water supply. One investigator reviewed the maps and tables from a preliminary version of the SCCMDP to screen for excessive bone cancer mortality in counties and states known to have high fluoride levels. No obvious associations were found. Data from the SCCMDP, which were obtained in a matter of minutes, provided important additional evidence that an association between bone cancer and fluoride does not seem to exist.

POINT OF DEPARTURE

POINT OF DEPARTURE

Tables 9-5 and 9-6
Rhode Island Breast Cancer Mortality, All Females, 1983-87
Examples of state summary tables showing different rank orders for the same data

Table 9-5
County breast cancer mortality ranked by rate

Rate	Error*		Exposed**	Obsvd+	Exptd++	SMR#	County name	FIP##
2.24	8.71	-	122,201	55	46.2	119.0	Bristol	001
5.04	5.19	h	410,876	192	149.1	128.7	Kent	003
4.24	7.30	-	213,167	90	72.3	124.5	Newport	005
8.84	2.39	-	1,540,327	641	600.2	106.8	Providence	007
4.45	7.28	-	251,737	93	76.3	121.8	Washington	009

	United States		Rhode Island
Exposed:	613,087,040		2,538,308
Obsvd:	198,967		1,971
Rate:	27.16		30.81
Error:	0.12		1.95 (1.96 sd)

Table 9-6

County breast cancer mortality ranked by observed deaths (United States and Rhode Island data omitted)

Rate	Error*		Exposed**	Obsvd+	Exptd++	SMR#	County name	FIP##
28.84	2.39	-	1,540,327	641	600.2	106.8	Providence	007
35.04	5.19	h	410,876	192	149.1	128.7	Kent	003
34.45	7.28	-	251,737	93	76.3	121.8	Washington	009
34.24	7.30	-	213,167	90	72.3	124.5	Newport	005
32.24	8.71	-	122,201	55	46.2	119.0	Bristol	001

*   ± 1.96 standard deviations from rate.

**   Person years of exposure.

+   Number of deaths during time of observation (1983-1987).

++   Expected number of deaths if county rate was the same as the national rate.

\#   Observed deaths/expected deaths.

\#\#   Standard code for county within the state.

h   Counties with statistically high rates (confidence intervals do not overlap).

POINT OF DEPARTURE

P O I N T

O F

D E P A R T U R E

The National Cancer Institute (NCI) has distributed the SCCMDP program to the state health departments in the 48 coterminous states and the District of Columbia, and also to the Comprehensive Cancer Centers supported by the NCI. The CDC and the American Cancer Society are developing educational and support material for the program and will distribute the program through their networks throughout the United States. Arrangements to make the program available to a wider audience are under consideration. Those interested in additional information should contact their state health departments.

Table 9-7
Lung cancer mortality in Wilson County, North Carolina:
All Males, 40-85+, by pentad, 1953-1987

Number of Deaths

Age Group	1953-57	1958-62	1963-67	1968-72	1973-77	1978-82	1983-87	TOTAL
40-44	1	0	1	3	0	6	3	14
45-49	2	1	8	3	4	7	6	31
50-54	2	2	7	10	13	11	4	49
55-59	3	5	11	13	9	18	16	75
60-64	2	5	4	11	23	23	30	98
65-69	2	2	9	14	20	26	26	102
70-74	0	1	6	7	13	31	30	89
75-79	0	0	6	4	6	10	20	47
80-84	1	0	0	2	1	4	3	11
85-up	0	0	0	0	2	3	4	9
Total	13	21	52	67	91	139	142	525

Age-Adjusted Rates

| ADJST | 38.1 | 57.5 | 130.1 | 157.0 | 204.1 | 291.2 | 273.9 | 182.6 |

POINT OF DEPARTURE

Technical Notes

Map Design and Construction:
General Issues

The maps included in this book provide a means of emphasizing and graphically depicting a variety of spatial techniques. Our practice was to follow standard cartographic conventions of map design. A superior map requires a considerable amount of planning; a thoughtful consideration of the elements involved in map design encompasses compilation, generalization, layout, and data evaluation. Compilation requires securing source materials, preparing a worksheet or rough draft(s) showing the arrangement of all elements for inclusion on the final map, and compiling information in a specification sheet which includes such information as line weights and styles (e.g., dashed or solid). Generalization is the process of selecting, simplifying, or combining the information to facilitate the optimal cartographic representation of the data. Layout consists of organizing the five basic map elements: border, title, legend, scale bar, and north arrow. In some instances, particularly with thematic maps, the border scale bar and north arrow are optional as these may often be understood within context. Balance is also an issue of concern during the layout process. The base map (map outline) together with the five basic elements should be positioned for balance or symmetry with respect to each other in the given space. However, an informal design using nonsymmetrical balance is acceptable in situations where such a design is appropriate. For instance, the maps and graphics in *USA Today* represent non-traditional uses of cartography, many of which are representationally incorrect although dramatic. For clarity and accuracy, consistency in content and in scale are vital since it is just as possible to "lie with maps" as it is to "lie with statistics" (Monmonier M. 1991. *How to lie with maps*. Chicago: University of Chicago Press). Cartographers operating within a department or organizational unit may want to standardize the five basic elements for consistency and to avoid misrepresentation of data.

The cartographer is responsible for evaluating the data set to determine its level of measurement and then selecting a classification method. There are four common levels of measurement for most data: nominal, ordinal, interval, and ratio. Data manipulation and classification commence following determination of the appropriate level of measurement. Sometimes this involves using descriptive statistics such as the mean, median, or mode of the variable under consideration (e.g., median income by county). Other classification methods include: classifying by equal steps (find the range of the data set and divide by the desired number of classes), quantiles (each class has the same number of observations), natural breaks (subjective interpretation of class limits usually determined by plotting data values on graph paper and looking for natural breaks), and minimum variance method (the intra-class variance is minimized while the inter-class variance is maximized). These alternative approaches vary in their utility and appropriateness and are available within most software packages and described in general cartography texts. The choice of data breaks in a distribution is very subjective and resultant representations of data may vary quite substantially, depending on the classification method chosen. We suggest that multiple alternative classification methods be tried out and the results compared so that the final map depicts the data not only accurately, but optimally and appropriately.

Production of the Handbook

The current application of geographic techniques to health services research involves the use of increasingly complex computer programs and very sophisticated hardware. The development of this book is an example of the use of multiple operating systems, software packages and various machine configurations. The editorial team and the authors of the chapters made use of many different commercially available products to illustrate the techniques discussed and to bring the final document to publication.

The final text and illustrations for the book have been produced using Pagemaker® versions 4.2a and 5.0. The text and graphics were processed on a Macintosh IIfx, Macintosh IIcx, and Macintosh Centris 650, using 20,8, and 24 megabytes of internal memory respectively, with operating systems 6.4, 7.0.1 and 7.1. Since software and operating systems evolve so rapidly, there have been multiple changes in versions of the operating system as well as the application software packages used in this book. The camera-ready pages were imaged on an Apple LaserWriter Pro 630 at 600 dots per inch and used by University Press of America for final page make-up.

To create maps used in the text, the authors and the cartographers working on the book used several packages, mostly working within the Macintosh environment although occasionally maps were created originally in a DOS or Windows environment. We make reference to full-size GIS systems, and the authors from the Department of Geography at the University of North Carolina at Chapel Hill (UNC-CH) made use of the ARC/INFO system installed at the Geography Department. This system is mounted on SUN workstations, using the UNIX operating system, with 48-64 megabytes of internal memory per workstation. Data sets for the mapping and analysis examples were generally manipulated on the mainframe computer at the University of North Carolina at Chapel Hill, which includes an IBM 3090-170 mainframe computer, several VAX 6330 minicomputers and a Convex C240 supercomputer. All of these are network-accessible and are maintained by the University of North Carolina at Chapel Hill's Office of Information Technology (OIT). The interface with the mainframe was through WYLBUR and most data sets were managed using the SAS® system.

Data sets were downloaded to mapping and graphics packages in text (ASCII) format and were occasionally manipulated using statistical packages such as Statview® or JMP® on microcomputers. Graphing of data was primarily done using DeltaGraph Professional®; the population pyramids were created using IPSS®. Final imaging for inclusion in Pagemaker format used Freehand®, Super-Paint®, and MacDraw II®. Maps were produced using MapInfo® versions 1.0 and 2.0, Atlas Mapmaker® version 4.5, Atlas Pro® version 1.0, and Geoquery®. MapInfo was used in both the Macintosh and Windows environments. The people who produce MapInfo and Atlas Pro offer training sessions nationwide and can arrange for customized training sessions for groups or individuals. Contact them through the customer service numbers listed at the end of this section.

Data from the US Bureau of the Census were obtained using CD-ROM disks and downloaded using FoxBase®. Some detailed maps were produced from TIGER line files (1990 version) and were transported into the graphics environment using TIGER Massage®.

Special datasets were used for some maps and analyses or were discussed in the chapters as potential sources for baseline maps or for basic levels of data to be used in GIS applications. These ranged from the generally applicable Census files such as the Summary Tape Files (STF) that include the entire US population and special samples of the population, to special use tapes and data sets including the AIDS Public Information Data Set available from the National Center for Infectious Disease, Centers for Disease Control and Prevention in Atlanta, Georgia.

There are thousands of data sets now in existence that could be used with hundreds of mapping applications, and the reader who may want to browse one of the more complete listings of these programs should refer to the *1993 International GIS Sourcebook* published by GIS World or review recent issues of *GIS World*, a monthly magazine aimed at the more complex system user.

The individual who would like to explore maps in more depth should consult *The Map Catalog, 3rd Edition: Newly Revised, Every Map and Chart on Earth and Even Some Above It*, published by Vintage Books. Another guide to the use of mapping that readers might find useful is *Analytical Mapping and Geographic Databases* by G. David Garson and Robert S. Biggs, published by Sage as part of their series on Quantitative Applications in the Social Sciences.

Doing it yourself is rewarding and challenging but also often frustrating; this holds for computer mapping. There are resources available at almost any department of geography in colleges and universities and you shouldn't overlook the opportunity to consult them if you need guidance to enter the field or to improve your skills.

Contact Information

Aldus FreeHand: Aldus Corporation, 411 First Avenue South, Seattle, WA 98104-2871; 206-628-2320.

Aldus PageMaker: Aldus Corporation, 411 First Avenue, Seattle, WA 98104-28711; 206-628-2320.

Atlas MapMaker or AtlasPro: Strategic Mapping, Inc., 4030 Moorpark Avenue, Suite 250, San Jose, CA 95117; 408-985-7400.

Aldus SuperPaint: Silicon Beach Software, Inc., a subsidiary of Aldus Corporation, 9880 Carroll Center Road, Suite J, San Diego, CA 99126-4551; 619-695-6959.

Delta Graph Professional: DeltaPoint, Inc., 2 Harris Court, Suite B-1, Monterey, CA 93940; 408-648-4000.

FoxBase+: Microsoft Corporation; 419-874-0162.

*GIS World***:** GIS World, Inc., 155 E. Boardwalk Drive, Suite 250, Fort Collins, CO 80525; 303-223-4848, fax: 303-223-5700.

GeoQuery: P.O. Box 206, Naperville, IL 60566; 708-357-0535.

IPSS: PSRC Software, Population and Society Research Center, Bowling Green, OH 43403; 419-372-2497.

JMP: SAS Institute Inc., SAS Campus Drive, Cary, NC 27513; 919-677-8000.

MacDraw Pro: Claris Corporation, 5201 Patrick Henry Drive, M/S C-70, Box 58168, Santa Clara, CA 95052-8168; 408-727-8227.

MapInfo: MapInfo Corporation, 200 Broadway, Troy, NY 12180; 800-327-8627.

StatView: Abacus Concepts, Inc., 1984 Bonita Avenue, Berkeley, CA 94704; 510-540-1949.

Glossary of Technical Terms

access: the ability to use a service or thing. In health care it may be "potential" indicating physical proximity or ability to use services, or "realized" indicating actual or effective use of services.

activity space: the limited geographic areas within which individuals typically live, work, shop, and seek services (e.g., health care, day care for children and elderly dependents, entertainment).

birth rate: the number of babies born in a given time period divided by the total population. Birth rates from small areas are usually combined for several years to provide a stable estimate of actual rates.

Cartesian or X- Y- coordinates: points in space are represented by Cartesian (x, y) coordinates; a line is referenced by a string of coordinates, and an area or polygon by a string of coordinates starting and ending at the same point.

cartography: the art and science of map making; the construction and design of maps.

central place theory: the hierarchical ordering of goods and services according to place size.

choropleth(ic) map: a map where appropriate area shadings (value, texture, intensity) are assigned to the regions for which information is collected prior to mapping (e.g., population density by county).

cluster: the grouping of similar objects whereby the scientist typically sets up rules for detection that circumvent a random occurrence of the grouping.

coefficient of localization: a single, summary number used to describe the relative concentration of an activity in a region.

commitment index: method of determining medical service area; the portion of a hospital's admissions from a given area.

core specialists: those physicians required to constitute a working medical community including: general and family practitioners, general pediatricians, general surgeons, general internal medicine physicians, and obstetricians and gynecologists.

crow-fly method: a technique used to determine relative distance between two points in space. *See* straight line distance.

demography or demographic: the scientific and statistical study of population—in particular, the size of populations and their development and structure.

difference map: mapping the difference between comparable variables, e.g., a map of the difference between the total number of children aged two and the number aged two with complete immunization.

dot map: point symbol(s) are used to show the form of the spatial distribution of some feature and its magnitude. Dots are the most common symbol but any other geometric figure—square, circle, or triangle—may be used. The shape is irrelevant since the meaning of the symbol lies in its repetition (e.g., each dot represents 25,000 people; divide total population by 25,000; the result is the number of dots to be placed). The aim is not to give precise locational information but rather to present an image of changing density from one region to the next.

demographic base map: a map for which the size of units is proportional to the numbers of people or resources rather than area.

demographic transition: describes a rapid change in the birth and/or death rates for a country or region undergoing development and an improvement in living conditions.

diffusion: the spread or movement outward from a point or beginning place, usually pertaining to disease, ideas, or innovations. Various types include: expansion, relocation, contagious, contact, and hierarchical. Innovations usually move very quickly to the top of the urban hierarchy (largest city or cities) and then cascade down; the diffusion of diseases is typically a combination such that an epidemic may follow a contagious pattern yet be affected by migration (relocation) and the hierarchical structuring of movement.

distance decay or friction of distance: is derived from the gravity model. As applied to health care, it typically measures the interactions between a single provider (clinician or facility) and people at varying distances from the resource. The friction of distance or how rapidly the interaction decreases as distance increases is usually displayed by means of a distance decay curve.

divergency graphs: line graphs illustrating different distributions.

ecological fallacy: arises when statistics or data are compared across scales, such that a state-level risk factor cannot be used to predict what will happen to specific individuals. (Similarly, one could not interview one individual and thereby make generalizations about a county or state population.) This means that patterns of association are different at different scales of analysis, and it is an error to take an association that is true at one scale and infer that it will be true at any other scale. However, observed associations at one scale can be used as clues to direct analyses at other levels of analysis.

epicenter: a major source area of disease transmission.

epidemic: any disease, infectious or chronic, occurring at a greater frequency than usually expected.

epidemiology: the study of the distribution and determinants of disease frequency in human populations.

etiology: the nature or study of disease causation.

fertility rate: the number of babies born in a given time period divided by the number of women of childbearing age (15-45 by convention), which is then commonly multiplied by 1,000.

flow map: a map depicting thematic data using proportional flow lines to portray the transportation of goods or people.

foci: the plural of focus.

friction of distance: the delays that increase travel time from one point to another due to intersections, urban congestion, road conditions, or speed limits.

geocodes: geographic references tying attribute data to some spatial element on the ground.

geography: the science of the earth's form and its physical divisions. In health services research geography is concerned with how human actions are affected by distance across the earth's surface and how humans interact to preserve or enhance health over distance.

geographic access: refers to the time and physical distance that must be traversed to get care, usually measured in distance or travel time from a person's residence to a source of care.

geographic information system (GIS): is defined as a computer-based system with a fundamental data structure that uses location as one of its essential elements. The major components of a GIS are computer hardware and a graphics output device, a set or sets of application software modules, and a dataset which includes geographic or spatially-referenced variables (e.g., by ZIP code, x- y-coordinate, county).

geopolitical boundary: a border set up for governmental purposes (e.g., counties, tax districts, boroughs).

Gini coefficient(s): the most common summary measure of inequality, usually used in conjunction with the Lorenz curve. It is defined as one minus the area between the Lorenz curve and the diagonal.

gravity model: a model of flow patterns derived from an analogy to the formula for gravity attraction which states that the attractional force between two objects is directly proportional to their masses and inversely proportional to the square of the distance between them.

human ecology: the ways human behavior, in its cultural and socioeconomic context, interacts with environmental conditions to produce or prevent disease among susceptible people.

incidence: quantifies the number of new events or cases of disease that develop in a population at risk during a specified time period.

index of dissimilarity: the most common summary measure of inequality which is used in conjunction with the Lorenz curve. It is defined graphically as the maximum vertical deviation between the Lorenz curve and the diagonal. (See **Gini coefficient**.)

latitude and longitude: a two-dimensional referencing system for navigation which measures, by degrees of arc, great circles of the globe running north/south and east/west.

location: position in two-dimensional space.

location quotient: an index for comparing an area's share of a particular activity with the area's share of some basic or aggregate phenomenon.

Logit model: a regression model in which the dependent variable is categorical versus continuous such that it can take on a limited number of values (e.g., yes/no, white/black/other, high/low) and through transformation can be estimated within the standard OLS methodology.

Lorenz curve: a divergency graph showing the differences between two accumulating distributions. It is commonly used to measure the extent of inequality of a variable distributed over aspatial categories.

macro-micro scales: the scale of analysis where *macro* refers to the study of populations over relatively large areas, versus *micro* which refers to individuals confined to smaller, more local areas.

map: a geographic image of the environment; a geographical picture or snapshot that can display features or characteristics of an area.

maximum likelihood (ML): a mathematical method of point estimation with some stronger theoretical properties than the method of ordinary least squares.

medical geography: is both an ancient perspective and relatively new specialty, using the graphical techniques and tools of geography to analyze health care issues. It encompasses health issues related to the spatial variation of resources as well as disease ecology.

migration: movement across a political boundary with the intent of permanent change of residence.

Minkowski Metric: measures distance between two points, but includes a factor that can be adjusted for perceptual differences (see page 99 for mathematical formula).

mobility: movement of people, including migration and circulation across all scales of time and distance.

morbidity: sickness or state of being diseased.

morbidity rate: the incidence rate of nonfatal cases in the total population at risk during a specified period of time. For example, the morbidity rate of tuberculosis in 1990 can be calculated by dividing the number of incident cases in 1990 by the midyear population.

mortality: death.

mortality rate: the incidence of death in a particular population during a given period of time, calculated by dividing the number of deaths during the stated time period by the total population. It can be calculated for both total mortality or for cause-specific mortality.

MSAs: medical service areas; geographic distance, geopolitical boundaries, and patient origin are some approaches to medical service area delineation. (MSA may also indicate Metropolitan Statistical Area.)

nephrosis: any disease of the kidney.

observed-to-expected ratio: the number of observed cases of a disease divided by the number of expected cases, calculated using an indirect standardization procedure.

odds ratio: ratio of the odds of exposure among cases to those among the controls in an epidemiologic study.

oncology: the study of tumors, typically cancerous or malignant.

ordinary least squares (OLS): the most commonly used mathematical method of regression analysis, which minimizes the sum of the squared errors in estimating parameters.

overlay map: integrating spatial information from separate map areas of coverage.

population density: a measure of the dispersion of the population over an area whereby total population is divided by land area.

population potential: a measure of population distribution that describes the nearness or accessibility of people to a point location by summarizing location relative to the location of all surrounding populations. In geographic terms, density is a site measure while potential is a measure of situation.

population pyramid: a graphical display of the age and sex structure of a population.

prevalence: the proportion of individuals in a population who have a disease at a specific point in time.

primary care: prevention of disease and the care of uncomplicated, common illnesses, usually provided by family physicians, general internists, and pediatricians. Some specialists provide substantial amounts of primary care to specific populations, e.g., obstetricians and gynecologists.

proportion: a type of ratio where those who are included in the numerator must also be included in the denominator (e.g., the proportion of women over the age of 50 who have had a hysterectomy). It is expressed as a percentage.

rate: a ratio in which there is a distinct relationship between the numerator and the denominator and a measure of time is intrinsically part of the denominator (e.g., the number of newly diagnosed cases of breast cancer per 100,000 women during a given year). Rates give the frequency of one event relative to another within a given period of time.

ratio: a general term that includes a number of more specific measures such as: proportion, percentage, and rate. Ratios describe the proportion of one absolute quantity as compared to another at a given point in time (e.g., total population to number of physicians).

regionalization: the careful, planned allocation of health care resources, usually based on a tiered structure (e.g., hierarchical) of facilities and/or providers linked by established referral networks.

relevance index: method of determining medical service area; the proportion of an area's admissions accounted for by a given hospital.

replacement reproduction: producing the number of children needed to replace the adult parents, usually considered in developed countries to be 2:1 since not every girl conceived lives to reproduce.

road distance: a measure of relative distance that takes into account the route taken from some referent point to a designated destination (e.g., residence to provider).

rural: a concept that describes people, places, and things. Usually associated with less dense population and agricultural activity, it is a complex and multifaceted idea. Not urban, in the US Census definition.

scale: the defined dimensional relationship between reality and a map where small scale refers to large areas (1:100,000,000) and large scale refers to smaller areas (1:75,000).

scale of analysis: the size of the area under consideration (e.g., county level, state level).

SDE: standard deviational ellipse; technique of summarizing point patterns with ellipses; graphic representation of average location, dispersion, and orientation of point data in x-y coordinate space.

seropositive: showing positive results on serological examination.

service area: the geographic area from which people use a particular health care provider.

spatial: pertaining to space.

standardization of rates: a statistically constructed adjustment of rates that takes into account the difference between populations with respect to other variables of interest (e.g., race, age, sex). There are two types of standardization: 1) the indirect method, and 2) the direct method.

state plane coordinate systems: one or more referencing grids devised by the US Geological Survey for mapping each state. These grids minimize distortion from flattening the curvature of the earth and are widely used for urban and regional mapping.

straight line distance or linear distance or map distance: is the measured distance between two points on a map. It is commonly used because it is both quick and relatively easy to determine.

temporal: having to do with time or time trends.

tertiary care: higher order, specialized medical services (e.g., oncology, burn units, trauma centers).

time distance or travel time: the time it takes to travel between two points.

urban: a concept of place and people associated with high population density and complex social systems. Specific definitions are based on the identification of boundable places that identify social action spaces.

urology: the branch of medicine that concerns itself with the urinary tract in both sexes and the genital organs in males.

utilization: revealed accessibility or the measurable number of services used such as number of outpatient visits or number of inpatient admissions.

vector: a carrier, especially the animal (usually an arthropod) which transfers an infective agent from one host to another.

vector analysis: a cartographic technique using arrows to represent both magnitude and direction of movement of some phenomenon (see also **flow map**).

References

CHAPTER 1 INTRODUCTION

Cliff AD, and P Haggett. 1988. *Atlas of disease distributions: Analytic approaches to epidemiological data.* Oxford, UK: Basil Blackwell.

Jusatz HL, ed. 1952-. *World atlas of epidemic diseases.* Hamburg, Germany: Falk-Verlag.

May JM. 1958. *The ecology of human disease.* New York: MD Publications.

Meade MS, JW Florin, and WM Gesler. 1988. *Medical geography.* New York: The Guilford Press.

CHAPTER 2 FOCUS ON RURAL AND REGIONAL HEALTH CARE DELIVERY

Area Resource File (ARF). 1992. Office of Data Analysis and Management, Bureau of Health Professions, US Department of Health and Human Services; March.

Austin CM, Honey R, and Eagle TC. 1987. *Human geography.* St. Paul, MN: West Publishing Company.

Baldwin DC, and B Rowley. 1990. Alternative models for the delivery of rural health care: A case study of a western frontier state. *Journal of Rural Health* 6(3):256-272.

Bronstein JM. 1992. Entrance and exit of obstetrics providers in rural Alabama. *Journal of Rural Health* 8(2):114-120.

Budetti PP. 1984. The 'trickle-down' theory—Is that any way to make policy? *American Journal of Public Health* 74(12):1303-1304.

Butler M. 1990. *Rural-urban continuum codes for metro and nonmetro counties.* Washington DC: Economic Research Service, US Department of Agriculture.

Clifford WB, MK Miller, and CS Stokes. 1986. Rural-urban differences in mortality in the United States, 1970-1980. In: *New dimensions in rural policy: Building upon our heritage*, ed. D Jahr, W Johnson, RC Wimberly, pp. 63-70. Studies prepared for the Joint Economic Committee, US Congress. Washington, DC: US Government Printing Office.

Cordes S. 1989. The changing rural environment and the relationship between health services and rural development. *Health Services Research* 23(6):757-784.

Elison G. 1986. Frontier areas: Problems for delivery of health care services. *Rural Health Care* 8(5):1, 3.

Establishment of criteria for determining priorities among designated health professional shortage areas. 1991. *Federal Register* 56(161):41363-41365, August 20.

Frenzen PD. 1991. The increasing supply of physicians in US urban and rural areas, 1975 to 1988. *American Journal of Public Health* 81(9):1141-1147.

Fruen MA, and JR Cantwell. 1982. Geographic distribution of physicians: Past trends and future influences. *Inquiry* 19(1):44-50.

Hewitt M. 1989. *Defining "rural" areas: Impact on health care policy and research*. US Office of Technology Assessment Staff Paper. Washington, DC: US Government Printing Office.

Hewitt M. 1992. Defining "rural" areas: Impact on health care policy and research. In: *Health in rural North America: The geography of health care services and research*, ed. WM Gesler and TC Ricketts, pp. 25-54. New Brunswick, NJ: Rutgers University Press.

Hong W, and DA Kindig. 1992. The relationship between commuting patterns and health resources in nonmetropolitan counties of the United States. *Medical Care* 30(12):1154-58.

Jeffers JR, MF Bognanno, and JC Bartlett. 1971. On the demand versus need for medical services and the concept of "shortage." *American Journal of Public Health* 61(1):46-63.

Joint Task Force of the National Association of Community Health Centers and the National Rural Health Association. 1989. Health care in rural America: The crisis unfolds. *Journal of Public Health Policy* 10(1):99-116.

Kindig DA, and H Movassaghi. 1989. The adequacy of physician supply in small rural counties. *Health Affairs* 8(2):63-76.

Kindig DA, JR Schmelzer, and W Hong. 1992. Age distribution and turnover of physicians in nonmetropolitan counties of the United States. *Health Services Research* 27(4):565-578.

Kriesberg HM, et al. 1976. Prepared by Nathan Associates; edited by Aspen Systems Corporation. *Methodological approaches for determining health manpower supply and requirements, Volume II: Practical planning manual.* DHEW Contract No. HRA 230-75-0067; DHHS Publication No. (HRA) 76-14512.

Madison DL, and CD Combs. 1981. Location patterns of recent physician settlers in rural America. *Journal of Community Health* 6(4):267-274.

Marx L. 1964. *The machine in the garden: Technology and the pastoral ideal in America.* New York: Oxford University Press.

McGranahan DA, JC Hession, FK Hines, and MF Jordan. 1986. *Social and economic characteristics of the population in metro and nonmetro counties, 1970-80.* Agriculture and Rural Economics Division, Economic Research Service, US Department of Agriculture. Rural Development Research Report No. 58.

Miller MK, and AE Luloff. 1981. Who is rural? A typological approach to the examination of rurality. *Rural Sociology* 46:608-25.

Monroe AC, TE Aldrich, TC Ricketts, and MR Cooper. 1992. *Proximity to state-of-the-art cancer care and stage at diagnosis: North Carolina, 1988.* Chapel Hill, NC: North Carolina Rural Health Research Program, Cecil G. Sheps Center for Health Services Research.

Mullner RM, and D McNeil. 1986. Rural and urban hospital closures: A comparison. *Health Affairs* 5(3):131-141.

Mullner RM, RJ Rydman, DG Whiteis, and RF Rich. 1989. Rural community hospitals and factors correlated with their risk of closing. *Public Health Reports* 104(4):315-325.

National Rural Health Association (NRHA). 1991. Statement of the National Rural Health Association Board of Directors in deposition to US District Court. Washington, DC.

Newhouse JP, AP Williams, BW Bennett, and WB Schwartz. 1982. Where have all the doctors gone? *Journal of the American Medical Association* 247(17):2392-2396.

Newhouse JP. 1990. Geographic access to physician services. *Annual Review of Public Health* 11:207-230.

New York State Legislative Commission on Rural Resources. 1990. *Training physicians for rural health careers in New York State*. Albany, NY: New York State Legislature.

No more frontier? 1993. *Census and You* 28(7):9.

Patton L. 1989. Setting the rural health services research agenda: The Congressional perspective. *Health Services Research* 23(6):1006-1051.

Pickard J. 1988. A new county classification system. *Appalachia* 21(3):19-24, Summer.

Popper FJ. 1986. The strange case of the contemporary American frontier. *Yale Review* 76(1):101-21.

Pratt DS. 1990. Occupational health and the rural worker: Agriculture, mining, and logging. *Journal of Rural Health* 6(4):399-417.

Ricketts TC, and D Pathman. 1991. Review of methodology for needs assessment and health personnel projections in rural health. In: *Primary care research: Theory and methods*, ed. H Hibbard, PA Nutting, and ML Grady, pp. 239-251. Rockville, MD: Agency for Health Care Policy and Research. AHCPR Publication No. 91-0011.

Rowles GD. 1988. What's rural about rural aging? An Appalachian perspective. *Journal of Rural Studies* 4(2):115-124.

Schwartz WB, JP Newhouse, BW Bennett, AP Williams. 1980. The changing geographic distribution of board-certified physicians. *New England Journal of Medicine* 303(18):1032-1038.

Study of models to meet rural health care needs through mobilization of health professions education and services resources. 1992. Prepared for the Health Resources and Services Administration, Contract No. HRSA-240-89-0037.

US Bureau of Health Manpower. 1977. *Review of health manpower requirements standards.* Rockville, MD. HRA 77-22.

US Office of Technology Assessment (OTA). 1990. *Health care in rural America.* Washington, DC: US Government Printing Office. OTA-H-434.

Wibberly GP. 1972. Conflicts in the countryside. *Town and Country Planning* 40:259-64.

Williams AP, WB Schwartz, JP Newhouse, and BW Bennett. 1983. How many miles to the doctor? *New England Journal of Medicine* 309(16):958-963.

Willits FK, RC Bealer, and VL Timbers. 1990. Popular images of "rurality": Data from a Pennsylvania survey. *Rural Sociology* 55(4):559-578.

CHAPTER 3   CHANGES AND MEASURES IN THE CRUCIAL
            DIMENSION OF POPULATION

Bennett DG. 1990. *The impact of elderly in-migration on private and public economic development efforts in predominantly rural areas along the South Atlantic coast.* Report to the US Department of Commerce, Economic Development Administration. EDA Project No. 99-07-13732.

Brown DL, and CL Beale. 1981. Diversity in post-1970 population trends. In: *Nonmetropolitan America in transition*, ed. AH Hawley and SM Mazie, pp. 27-71. Chapel Hill, NC: University of North Carolina Press.

Cefalo RC, and G Gay. 1988. Standard terminology for reporting of reproductive health statistics in the United States. *Public Health Reports* 103(5):464-471.

DuMouchel WH, and GJ Duncan. 1983. Using sample survey weights in multiple regression analyses of stratified samples. *Journal of the American Statistical Association* 78(383):535-543.

Forstall RL. 1991. *Regional and metropolitan/nonmetropolitan population trends in the United States, 1980-90.* Paper presented to the Association of American Geographers, Miami, Florida, April 14, 1991 (revised Nov. 13, 1991).

Fry JD, and W Young. 1992. *The health care data source book; Finding the right information and making the most of it.* American Hospital Association. Chicago, IL: American Hospital Publishing.

Kiecolt KJ, and LE Nathan. 1985. *Secondary analysis of survey data.* Beverly Hills, CA: Sage Publications.

Korn EL, and BI Graubard. 1991. Epidemiologic studies utilizing surveys: Accounting for the sampling design. *American Journal of Public Health* 81(9):1166-1173.

Landis JR, JM Lepkowski, A Eklund, and SA Stenhouwer. 1982. Statistical methodology for analyzing data from a complex survey: The first national health and nutrition examination survey. *Vital and Health Statistics*, Series 2, No. 92. DHHS Publication No. 82-1366.

Lee ES, RN Forthofer, and RJ Lorimor. 1989. *Analyzing complex survey data.* Quantitative Series No. 07-071. Newbury Park: Sage Publications.

Lichter DT, GV Fuguitt, and TB Heaton. 1985. Components of nonmetropolitan population change: The contributions of rural areas. *Rural Sociology* 50(1)88-98.

Long L. 1988. *Migration and residential mobility in the United States.* New York, NY: Russell Sage Foundation.

Meade MS. 1992. Implications of changing demographic structures for rural health services. In: *Health in rural North America: The geography of health care services and research*, ed. WM Gesler and TC Ricketts, pp. 69-85. New Brunswick, NJ: Rutgers University Press.

Meade MS, JW Florin, and WM Gesler. 1988. *Medical geography*. New York: The Guilford Press.

Morrill RL. 1988. Migration regions and population redistribution. *Growth and Change* 19: 43-60.

Morrill RL. 1993. Development, diversity, and regional demographic variability. *US Annals of the Association of American Geographers* 83(3):406-433.

North Carolina Center for Health and Environmental Statistics. 1991. *Detailed mortality statistics, 1990*. Raleigh, NC.

Raine JW. 1978. Summarizing point patterns with the standard deviational ellipse. *Area* 10: 328-333.

Stewart JQ, and W Warntz. 1958. Physics of population distribution. *Journal of Regional Science* 1:99-123.

US Bureau of the Census. 1991. Geographical mobility: March 1987 to March 1990. *Current Population Reports*, series P-20, No. 456. Washington, DC: US Government Printing Office.

US National Center for Health Statistics (US NCHS). 1991. Advance report of final natality statistics, 1989. *Monthly Vital Statistics Report* 40(8), supplement Dec.12, Table 3.

US National Center for Health Statistics (US NCHS). 1992. Births, marriages, divorce and deaths for 1991 (provisional data). *Monthly Vital Statistics Report* 40(12).

US National Center for Health Statistics (US NCHS). 1992. *Catalog of electronic data products from the National Center for Health Statistics*. Washington, DC: US Government Printing Office. DHHS Publication No. (PHS) 92-1213.

US National Center for Health Statistics (US NCHS). 1993. *Health, United States, 1992*. Hyattsville, MD: Public Health Service.

US National Institute of Mental Health. 1989. *Small area analysis: Estimating total population.* Rockville, MD.

Yuill RS. 1971. The standard deviational ellipse: An updated tool for spatial description. *Geografiska Annaler* 53B: 28-39.

CHAPTER 4   ACCESS TO HEALTH SERVICES

Aday L, and R Andersen. 1974. A framework for the study of access to medical care. *Health Services Research* 9(3):208-220.

Aday L, R Andersen, and GV Fleming. 1980. *Health care in the US: Equitable for whom?* Beverly Hills, CA: Sage Publications.

Aday L, and R Andersen. 1975. *Access to medical care.* Ann Arbor, MI: Health Administration Press.

Andersen R, J Kravits, and OW Anderson. 1975. *Equity in health services: Empirical analyses in social policy.* Cambridge, MA: Ballinger Publishing Company.

Anderson R, and JF Newman. 1973. Societal and individual determinants of medical care utilization in the United States. *Milbank Memorial Fund Quarterly* 51:95-124, Winter.

Applebaum W. 1966. Methods for determining store trade areas, marketing penetration, and potential sales. *Journal of Marketing Research* 3:127-141, May.

Billings J. 1990. *Consideration of the use of small area analysis as a tool to evaluate barriers to access.* Paper prepared for the second HRSA Primary Care Conference on Education of Physicians to Improve Access to Care for the Underserved, Columbia, MD: March 21-23.

Centers for Disease Control. 1994. Vaccination coverage of 2-year-old children: United States, 1991-1992. *MMWR* 42(51-52).

Chassin MR. 1993. Explaining geographic variations: The enthusiasm hypothesis. *Medical Care* 31(5):YS37-YS44, supplement.

Codman Research Group. 1991. *Utilization of inpatient hopsital services by rural Medicare beneficiaries.* Prepared under contract to the Prospective Payment Assessment Commission. Technical Report No. E-91-03.

Committee on the Costs of Medical Care. 1972. *Medical care for the American people.* Final report, adopted October 31, 1932. New York: Arno Press and The New York Times (Reprint of 1932 Edition from University of Chicago Press).

Cowper PA, and JE Kushman. 1987. A spatial analysis of primary health care markets in rural areas. *American Journal of Agricultural Economics* August:613-625.

Diehr P, K Cain, F Connell, and E Volinn. 1990. What is too much variation? The null hypothesis in small-area analysis. *Health Services Research* 24(6):741-71.

Donabedian A. 1973. *Aspects of medical care administration: Specifying requirements for health care.* Published for the Commonwealth Fund. Cambridge, MA: Harvard University Press, pp. 402-485.

Elison G. 1986. Frontier areas: Problems for delivery of health care services. *Rural Health Care* 8(5):1,3.

Francis AM, and JB Schneider. 1984. Using computer graphics to map origin-destination data describing health care delivery systems. *Social Science and Medicine* 18(5):405-420.

Freed GL, Bordley WC, and DeFriese GH. 1993. Childhood immunization programs: An analysis of policy issues. *Milbank Memorial Fund Quarterly* 71(1):65-96.

Fry J. 1971. Medical care in three societies. Common problems and dilemmas in the USSR, USA, and UK. *International Journal of Health Services* 1(2):121-33.

Garnick DW, HS Luft, HC Robinson, and J Tetreault. 1987. Appropriate measures of hospital market areas. *Health Services Research* 22(1):69-89.

Gesler WM, and J Cromartie. 1985. Studying spatial patterns of illness and hospital use in a central Harlem health district. *Journal of Geography* 84:211-216.

Ginzberg E. 1977. *The limits of health reform, the search for realism.* NY: Basic Books.

Girt JL. 1973. Distance to general medical practice and its effect on revealed ill-health in a rural environment. *The Canadian Geographer* 17(2):154-166.

Gogan JP, Luikart C, and Bacon TJ. 1979. *County/cluster analysis of physician/population ratios.* Presented at the annual meeting of the American Public Health Association, November 7.

Graduate Medical Education National Advisory Committee. 1980. *Geographic distribution report, Vol. III.* DHHS Publication No. (HRA) 81-653. Washington, DC: US Government Printing Office.

Gross PF. 1972. Urban health disorders, spatial analysis and the economics of health facility location. *International Journal of Health Services* 2(1):63-84.

Hewitt M. 1989. *Defining "rural" areas: Impact on health care policy and research.* US Office of Technology Assessment Staff Paper. Washington, DC: US Government Printing Office.

Huff DL. 1963. A probabilistic analysis of consumer spatial behavior. In: *Emerging concepts in marketing.* Proceedings of the Winter Conference of the American Marketing Association, ed. WS Decker, pp. 443-461. Chicago, IL: American Marketing Association.

Huff DL. 1966. A programmed solution for approximating an optimal retail location. *Land Economics* 42:293-303.

Hongvivatana, T. 1984. Data analysis: Social science perspective. In: *Evaluating primary health care in southeast Asia, proceedings of a regional seminar.* New Delhi: Regional Office, World Health Organization.

Hulka BS. 1978. Epidemiological applications to health services research. *Journal of Community Health* 4(2):140-149.

Joseph AE, and PR Bantock. 1982. Measuring potential physical accessibility to general practitioners in rural areas: A method and case study. *Social Science and Medicine* 16:85-90.

Joseph AE, and DR Phillips. 1984. *Accessibility and utilization, geographical perspectives on health care delivery.* New York: Harper & Row.

Joseph AE, and A Poyner. 1981. *The utilization of three public services in a rural Ontario township: An empirical evaluation of a conceptual framework.* Centre for Resources Development, Publication No. 107. Ontario: University of Guelph.

Kane RL. 1975. Vector resolution: A new tool in health planning. *Medical Care* 13(2):126-136.

Leape LL, RE Park, DH Solomon, MR Chassin, J Kosecoff, and RH Brook. 1990. Does inappropriate use explain small-area variations in the use of health care services? *Journal of the American Medical Association* 263(5):669-672.

Mayer JD. 1983. The distance behavior of hospital patients: A disaggregated analysis. *Social Science and Medicine* 17(12):819-827.

McConnel CE, and LA Tobias. 1986. Distributional change in physician manpower, United States, 1963-1980. *American Journal of Public Health* 76(6):638-642.

McGuirk MA, and FW Porrell. 1984. Spatial patterns of hospital utilization: The impact of distance and time. *Inquiry* 21:84-95.

Meade MS, JW Florin, and WM Gesler. 1988. *Medical geography.* New York: The Guilford Press.

Millman M, ed. 1993. *Access to health care in America.* Washington, DC: National Academy Press.

Morrill R, and RJ Earickson. 1966. *Hospital service areas: Distance of hospital from patient home.* Working Paper 1.5, Chicago Regional Hospital Study, December.

Morrill RL, and RJ Earickson. 1968. Variation in the character and use of Chicago area hospitals. *Health Services Research* 3(2):224-238.

Morrill RL, RJ Earickson, and P Rees. 1973. Factors influencing distances traveled to hospitals. *Economic Geography* 46(2):161-171.

Morrisey MA, FA Sloan, and J Valvona. 1988. Defining geographic markets for hospital care. *Law and Contemporary Problems* 51(2):165-194.

Morrow JS. 1977. Toward a more normative assessment of maldistribution: The Gini index. *Inquiry* 14:278-292.

Mountin JW, EH Pennell, and V Nicolay. 1942. Location and movement of physicians, 1923 and 1938; General observations. *Public Health Reports* 57(37):1363-75.

Muus KJ, and KA Ahmed. 1991. Physician utilization behavior among rural residents. *Focus on Rural Health* 8(2):10-12.

Northcutt HC. 1980. Convergence or divergence: The rural-urban distribution of physicians and dentists in Census divisions and incorporated cities, towns, and villages in Alberta, Canada 1956-1976. *Social Science and Medicine* 14D:17-22, 1980.

Patrick DL, J Stein, M Porta, CQ Porter, and TC Ricketts. 1988. Poverty, use of health services, and health status in rural america. *Milbank Memorial Fund Quarterly* 66(1):105-136.

Paul-Shaheen P, JD Clark, and D Williams. 1987. Small area analysis: A review and analysis of the North American literature. *Journal of Health Politics, Policy and Law* 12(4):741-809.

Penchansky R. 1976. Book review: Access to medical care. *Medical Care* 14(7):642.

Penchansky R. 1977. *The concept of access: A definition.* Unpublished report prepared for the National Health Planning Information Center, Bureau of Health Planning and Resource Development, Department of Health, Education and Welfare. Contract No. HRA 230-75-0073.

Penchansky R, and JW Thomas. 1981. The concept of access: Definition and relationship to consumer satisfaction. *Medical Care* 19(2):127-140.

Popper FJ. 1986. The strange case of the contemporary American frontier. *Yale Review* 76(1):101-21.

President's Commission for the Study of Ethical Problems in Medicine and Biomedical and Behavioral Research. 1983. *Securing access to health care: The ethical implications of differences in the availability of health services.* Volume One. Washington, DC: US Government Printing Office.

Rutstein DD, W Berenberg, TC Chalmers, CG Child, AP Fishman, and EB Perrin. 1976. Measuring the quality of medical care, a clinical method. *New England Journal of Medicine* 294(11):582-588.

Shannon G, J Lovett, and R Bashshur. 1979. Travel for primary care: Expectation and performance in a rural setting. *Journal of Community Health* 5(2):113-125.

Shannon GW, RL Bashshur, and CA Metzner. 1969. The concept of distance as a factor in accessibility and utilization of health care. *Medical Care Review* 26(2):143-161.

Shortell SM, TM Wickizer, and JRC Wheeler. 1984. Hospital-sponsored primary care: I. Organizational and financial effects. *American Journal of Public Health* 74(8):784-91.

Sneath PHA, and RR Sokal. 1973. *Numerical taxonomy, the principles and practice of numerical classification.* Chapters 1, 3, and 4. San Francisco, CA: WH Freeman and Company.

Study of models to meet rural health care needs through mobilization of health professions, education and services resources. 1992. Prepared for the Health Resources and Services Administration, Contract No. HRSA-240-89-0037.

Thouez JP, P Bodson, and AE Joseph. 1988. Some methods for measuring the geographic accessibility of medical services in rural regions. *Medical Care* 26(1):34-44.

US Department of Health and Human Services, Public Health Service. 1990. *Healthy people 2000, national health promotion and disease prevention objectives.* DHHS Publication No. (PHS) 91-50213.

Wennberg JE. 1984. Dealing with medical practice variations: A proposal for action. *Health Affairs* 3(2):6-32.

Wennberg JE. 1993. Future directions for small area variations. *Medical Care* 31(5):YS75-YS80, supplement.

Williams AP, WB Schwartz, JP Newhouse, and BW Bennett. 1983. How many miles to the doctor? *New England Journal of Medicine* 309(16):958-963.

Winter FW. 1986. Computerized secondary data approaches to health care location decisions. *Journal of Health Care Marketing* 6(2):67-75.

Wright GE. 1990. *Alternative hospital market area definitions.* Technical Report No. E-90-02. SysteMetrics/McGraw-Hill.

CHAPTER 5   HEALTH PROFESSIONS DISTRIBUTIONS

Barnett JR. 1987. Foreign medical graduates and the doctor shortage in New Zealand, 1973-1979. *New Zealand Medical Journal* 100(829):497-500.

Barnett JR. 1992. How long do general practitioners remain in any one location?: Regional and urban size variations in the turnover of foreign and New Zealand doctors in general practice, 1976-1990. *New Zealand Medical Journal* 105(933):169-171.

Chen MK. 1976. Two forms of an equity index for health resource allocation to minority groups. *Inquiry* 13:228-232.

Coulter PB. 1989. *Measuring inequality: A methodological handbook.* Boulder, CO: Westview Press.

Council on Graduate Medical Education (COGME). 1992. *Improving access to health care through physician workforce reform: Directions for the 21st century.* Rockville, MD: Health Resources and Services Administration.

Duncan OD, and B Duncan. 1955. A methodological analysis of segregation indexes. *American Sociological Review* 20:210-217.

Fein R. 1972. On achieving access and equity in health care. *Milbank Memorial Fund Quarterly* 50(4):157-190.

Gesler WM. 1992. Introduction. In: *Health in rural North America: The geography of health care services and delivery*, ed. WM Gesler and TC Ricketts. New Brunswick: Rutgers University Press.

Gober P, and RJ Gordon. 1980. Intraurban physician location: A case study of Phoenix. *Social Science and Medicine* 14D:407-417.

Greenberg MR. 1983. *Urbanization and cancer mortality*. New York: Oxford University Press.

Health Services Administration (HSA), Bureau of Community Health Services, Office of Monitoring and Analysis. 1973. *Background Paper: Health service scarcity area identification program*. August. Rockville, MD.

Health Services Research Group, University of Wisconsin. 1975. Development of an index of medical underservice. *Health Services Research* 10(2):168-180.

Horner RD, GP Samsa, and TC Ricketts. 1993. Preliminary evidence on retention rates of primary care physicians in rural and urban areas. *Medical Care* 31(7):640-648.

Isard W, and LN Moses. 1960. Interregional flow analysis and balance of payments statements. In: *Methods of regional analysis: An introduction to regional science*, ed. W Isard, pp. 122-81. Technology Press of the Massachusetts Institute of Technology and Wiley, New York.

Joseph AE. 1982. On the interpretation of the coefficient of localization. *Professional Geographer* 34(4):443-446.

Joseph AE, and PR Bantock. 1982. Measuring potential physical accessibility to general practitioners in rural areas: A method and case study. *Social Science and Medicine* 16(1): 85-90.

Joseph AE, and DR Phillips. 1984. *Accessibility and utilization: Geographical perspectives on health care delivery*. London: Harper & Row.

Kindig DA, and H Movassaghi. 1989. The adequacy of physician supply in small rural counties. *Health Affairs* (8)2:63-76.

Kindig DA, JR Schmelzer, and W Hong. 1992. Age distribution and turnover of physicians in nonmetropolitan counties of the United States. *Health Services Research* 27(4):565-78.

Kleinman JC, and RW Wilson. 1977. Are medically underserved areas medically underserved? *Health Services Research* 12(2):147-162.

Kletke PR, WD Marder, and AB Silberger. 1987. *The demographics of physician supply: Trends and projections.* Chicago, IL: AMA Center for Health Policy Research.

Kushman JE. 1977. The index of medical underservice as a predictor of ability to obtain physicians' services. *American Journal of Agricultural Economics* 59:192-197.

Lee RC. 1979. Designation of health manpower shortage areas for use by public health service programs. *Public Health Reports* 94(1):48-59.

Loft JD, and GA Ryan. 1985. *The American Medical Association's Physician Masterfile.* Proceedings of the 1985 Public Health Conference on Records and Statistics (USDHHS-PHS-NCHS), 86-1214, December. Hyattsville, MD.

Madison DL, and CD Combs. 1981. Location patterns of recent physician settlers in rural America. *Journal of Community Health* 6(4):267-274.

Marder WD, PR Kletke, AB Silberger, and RJ Willke. 1988. *Physician supply and utilization by specialty: Trends and projections.* Chicago, IL: AMA Center for Health Policy Research.

Monroe AC, Ricketts TC, and Savitz LA. 1992. Cancer in rural versus urban populations: A review. *Journal of Rural Health* 8(3):212-220.

Morrow JS. 1979. Commentary. Reply to Travis and Peters: A case of geographic 'normal mystique.' *Inquiry* 16(3):273-277.

Newhouse JP, AP Williams, BW Bennett, and WB Schwartz. 1982a. Where have all the doctors gone? *Journal of the American Medical Association* 247(17):2392-96.

Newhouse JP, AP Williams, BW Bennett, and WB Schwartz. 1982b. Does the geographical distribution of physician represent market failure? *Bell Journal of Economics* 3:493-502.

Newhouse JP, AP Williams, BW Bennett, and WB Schwartz. 1982c. *How have location patterns of physicians affected the availability of medical services?* Santa Monica: RAND Corporation.

NRHA helps defeat proposed rule reducing number of rural HMSAs. 1989. *Rural Health Care* 11(6):2.

Nutting PA, ed. 1987. *Community oriented primary care: From principle to practice.* Washington, DC: US Government Printing Office.

Pathman DE, TR Konrad, and TC Ricketts. 1992. The comparative retention of National Health Service Corps and other rural physicians. *Journal of the American Medical Association* 268(12):1552-1558.

Shortage area criteria. 1978. *Federal Register* 43(6):1586.

Shortage area criteria. 1978. *Federal Register* 43(137):30648.

Shortage area criteria. 1989. *Federal Register* 54(40):8735.

Shortage area criteria. 1990. *Federal Register* 55(126):27010.

Study of models to meet rural health care needs through mobilization of health professions education and services resources. 1992. Prepared for the Health Resources and Services Administration, Contract No. HRSA-240-89-0037.

Thouez JP, P Bodson, and AE Joseph. 1988. Some methods for measuring the geographic accessibility of medical services in rural regions. *Medical Care* 26(1):34-44.

US Bureau of Health Professions. 1980. *Evaluation of health manpower shortage area criteria.* DHEW Publication No.

344   *Geographic Methods for Health Services Research*

(HRA) 80-20. Rockville, MD: Health Resources and Services Administration.

US Bureau of Health Professions. 1983. *A report to Congress on the evaluation of health manpower shortage area criteria.* ODAM Reports No. 2-84. Rockville, MD: Health Resources and Services Administration.

US Bureau of Health Professions. 1992. *Division of Medicine UPDATE,* Spring. Rockville, MD: Health Resources and Services Administration.

US Department of Health and Human Services, Public Health Service. 1990. *Healthy people 2000, national health promotion and disease prevention objectives.* DHHS Publication No. (PHS) 91-50213.

US Division of Shortage Designation. 1993. *Selected statistics on health professional shortage areas as of September 30, 1993.* (Mimeo.) Bethesda, MD.

Williams AP, WB Schwartz, JP Newhouse, and BW Bennett. 1983. How many miles to the doctor? *The New England Journal of Medicine* 309(6):958-963.

Wright G. 1985. *Community characteristics and the competition for physicians in rural America, 1971-1981.* Report submitted to the Health Policy Division, Office of the Assistant Secretary for Planning and Evaluation, US DHHS. Contract No. 282-83-7300 to Macro Systems. Silver Spring, MD.

Wysong JA. 1975. The index of medical underservice: Problems in meaning, measurement, and use. *Health Services Research* 10:127-135.

CHAPTER 6   REGIONALIZATION OF HEALTH CARE

Anderson GM and J Lomas. 1989. Regionalization of coronary artery bypass surgery: Effects on access. *Medical Care* 27:288-296.

Antenucci JC, K Brown, PL Croswell, MJ Kevany, and H Archer. 1991. *Geographic information systems: A guide to the technology.* New York: Van Nostrand Reinhold.

Aronoff S. 1989. *Geographic information systems: A management perspective.* Ottawa: WDL Publications.

Berry BJ. 1964. Approaches to regional analysis: A synthesis. *Annals of the Association of American Geographers* 54(1): 2-11.

Campbell MK, GW Chance, R Natale, N Dodman, E Halinda, and L Turner. 1991. Is perinatal care in southwestern Ontario regionalized? *Canadian Medical Association Journal* 144(3):305-312.

Conover C, and M McLaughlin. 1991. Spreading the risk and beating the spread: The role of insurance in assuring adequate health care. *North Carolina Insight* 13:21-41.

Cowen DJ. 1990. GIS versus CAD versus DBMS: What are the differences? In: *Introductory readings in geographic information systems*, eds. DJ Peuquet and DF Marble, pp. 52-61. London: Taylor & Francis.

Elliott JP, DF O'Keeffe, and RK Freeman. 1982. Helicopter transportation of patients with obstetric emergencies in an urban area. *American Journal of Obstetrics and Gynecology* 143(2):157-162.

Finkler SA. 1979. Cost-effectiveness of regionalization: The heart surgery example. *Inquiry* 16(3):264-270.

Fiore BJ, LP Hanrahan, and HA Anderson. 1990. State health department response to disease cluster reports: A protocol for investigation. *American Journal of Epidemiology* 132(1 suppl):S14-22.

Florin JW. 1980. Health services regionalization in the United States. In: *Conceptual and methodological issues in medical geography,* ed. M Meade, pp. 282-298. Chapel Hill, NC: University of North Carolina at Chapel Hill, Studies in Geography No. 7.

Ginzberg E, ed. 1977. *Regionalization and health policy.* Washington, DC: US Department of Health, Education, and Welfare, Health Resources Administration, Publication No. 77-623.

Goldenberg RL. 1985. Vital statistics data as a measurement of perinatal regionalization in Alabama, 1970 to 1980. *Southern Medical Journal* 78:657-659.

Guthe WG, RK Tucker, EA Murphy, R England, E Stevenson, and JC Luckhardt. 1992. Reassessment of lead exposure in New Jersey using GIS technology. *Environmental Research* 59:318-325.

Harner EJ, and PB Slater. 1980. Identifying medical regions using hierarchical clustering. *Social Science and Medicine* 14D:3-10.

Harris G. 1991. A dearth of doctors in North Carolina—urban and rural. *North Carolina Insight* 13:76-88.

Hein HA. 1977. Regionalization of perinatal care in rural areas based on Iowa experience. *Seminars in Perinatology* 1:241-254.

International City Management Association. 1991. *The local government guide to geographic information systems: Planning and implementation.* Washington, DC: Public Technology Inc., and International City Management Association.

Lam NS. 1986. Geographical patterns of cancer mortality in China. *Social Science and Medicine* 23(3): 241-247.

Lambrew JM, and J Betts. 1991. Rural health care in North Carolina: Unmet needs, unanswered questions. *North Carolina Insight* 13:67-77.

Luft HS, JP Bunker, and AC Enthoven. 1979. Should operations be regionalized? *New England Journal of Medicine* 301(25):1364-69.

Maerki SC, HS Luft, and SS Hunt. 1986. Selecting categories of patients for regionalization. *Medical Care* 24(2):148-158.

Makuc DM, B Haglund, DD Ingram, JC Kleinman, and JJ Feldman. 1991. The use of health service areas for measuring provider availability. *Journal of Rural Health* 7(4) suppl:347-356.

Martin D. 1991. *Geographic information systems and their socioeconomic applications.* London: Routledge.

Matthews SA. 1990. Epidemiology using a GIS: The need for caution. *Computer, Environment and Planning* 17(16):213-221.

Mayfield JA, RA Rosenblatt, LM Baldwin, J Chu, JP Logerfo. 1990. The relation of obstetrical volume and nursery level to perinatal mortality. *American Journal of Public Health* 80(7):819-823.

McClafferty S, and D Broe. 1990. Patient outcomes and regional planning of coronary care services: A location-allocation approach. *Social Science and Medicine* 30(3):297-304.

Meyer HB. 1980. Regional care for mothers and their infants. *Clinical Perinatology* 7(1):205-221.

Navarro V. 1970. Methodology on regional planning of personal health services: A case study: Sweden. *Medical Care* 8(5):386-394.

Parr DM, ed. 1991. *Introduction to geographic information systems workshop.* Wilmington, NC: The Urban and Regional Information Systems Association.

Ricketts TC, ed. 1991. *National rural health policy atlas.* Chapel Hill, NC: Rural Health Research Program, Health Services Research Center, University of North Carolina at Chapel Hill.

Ross A, and S Davis. 1990. Point pattern analysis of the spatial proximity of residences prior to diagnosis of persons with Hodgkin's Disease. *American Journal of Epidemiology* 132:S53-S61.

Stallones L, JR Nuckols, and BK Berry. 1992. Surveillance around hazardous waste sites: Geographic information systems and reproductive outcomes. *Environmental Research* 59:81-92.

Star J, and J Estes. 1990. *Geographic information systems: An introduction.* Englewood Cliff, NJ: Prentice Hall.

Taylor DRF, ed. 1991. *Geographic information systems: The microcomputer and modern cartography.* Oxford, UK: Pergamon Press.

Tomich PG, and CL Anderson. 1990. Analysis of a maternal transport service within a perinatal region. *American Journal of Perinatology* 7:13-17.

Twigg L. 1990. Health based geographical information systems: Their potential examined in the light of existing data sources. *Social Science and Medicine* 30(1):143-155.

Verhasselt Y. 1993. Geography of health: Some trends and perspectives. *Social Science and Medicine* 36(2):119-123.

Walter SD, and SE Birnie. 1991. Mapping mortality and morbidity patterns: An international comparison. *International Journal of Epidemiology* 20:678-689.

Wartenberg D. 1992. Screening for lead exposure using a geographic information system. *Environmental Research* 59:310-317.

Zwarenstein M, D Krige, and B Wolff. 1991. The use of a geographical information system for hospital catchment area research in Natal/KwaZulu. *South Africa Medical Journal* 80:467-500.

CHAPTER 7   APPROACHES USED IN IDENTIFYING SERVICE
            AREAS

Dear M. 1977. Locational factors in the demand for mental health care. *Economic Geography* 53(3):223-240.

Diehr P, K Cain, F Connell, and E Volinn. 1990. What is too much variation? The null hypothesis in small-area analysis. *Health Services Research* 24(6):742-771.

Folland S, and M Stano. 1990. Small area variations: A critical review of propositions, methods, and evidence. *Medical Care Review* 47(4):419-465.

Garnick DW, HS Luft, JC Robinson, and J Tetreault. 1987. Appropriate measures of hospital market areas. *Health Services Research* 22(1):69-89.

Goody B. 1993a. Defining rural hospital markets. *Health Services Research* 28(2):183-200.

Goody B. 1993b. Sole providers of hospital care in rural areas. *Inquiry* 30(34):34-40.

Griffith JR. 1972. Determining population service areas and calculating use rates. *Quantitative techniques for hospital planning and control.* Lexington, MA: Lexington Books.

Griffith JR, JD Restuccia, PJ Tedeschi, PA Wilson, and HS Zuckerman. 1981. Measuring community hospital services in Michigan. *Health Services Research* 16(2):135-173.

Holahan J, RA Berenson, and PG Kachavos. 1990. Area variations in selected medicare procedures. *Health Affairs* 9(4):166-175.

Humphrey AB, and JS Buechner. 1992. Hospital service areas and utilization rates in a complex market. *The 1990's: A decade of decisions for vital and health statistics.* Washington, DC; July 1991. Hyattsville, MD: National Center for Health Statistics. (PHS) 92-1214:497-502.

Lubin JW, DL Drosness, and LG Wylie. 1965. Highway network minimum path selection applied to health facility planning. *Public Health Reports* 80(9):771-775.

Luft HS, and SC Maerki. 1984-85. Competitive potential of hospitals and their neighbors. *Contemporary Policy Issues* 3(2):89-102.

Makuc D, JC Kleinman, and MB Pierre Jr. 1985. Service areas for ambulatory medical care. *Health Services Research* 20(1):1-17.

Mayhew LD, RW Gibberd, and H Hall. 1986. Predicting patient flows and hospital case-mix. *Environment and Planning* 18(5):619-638.

McLafferty S. 1988. Predicting the effect of hospital closure on hospital utilization patterns. *Social Science and Medicine* 27(3):255-62.

Meade JA. 1974. A mathematical model for deriving hospital service areas. *International Journal of Health Services* 4(2):353-364.

Meade MS, JW Florin, and WM Gesler. 1988. *Medical geography*. New York: The Guilford Press.

Morrill RL, and R Earickson. 1968. Hospital variation and patient travel distances. *Inquiry* 5(4):26-34.

Morrill RL, and R Earickson. 1969. Locational efficiency of Chicago hospitals: An experimental model. *Health Services Research* 4(2):128-141.

Morrisey MA, FA Sloan, and J Valvona. 1988. Defining geographic markets for hospital care. *Law and Contemporary Problems* 51(2):165-194.

Pasley B, P Vernon, G Gibson, M McCauley, and J Andoh. 1987. Geographic variations in elderly hospital and surgical discharge rates, New York State. *American Journal of Public Health* 77(6):679-684.

Paul-Shaheen P, JD Clark, and D Williams. 1987. Small area analysis: A review and analysis of the North American literature. *Journal of Health Politics, Policy and Law* 12(4):741-809.

Phibbs CS, and JC Robinson. 1993. A variable-radius measure of local hospital market structure. *Health Services Research* 28(3):313-324.

Shannon GW, RL Bashshur, and CA Metzner. 1969. The concept of distance as a factor in accessibility and utilization of health care. *Medical Care Review* 26(2):143-160.

Stano M. 1993. Evaluating the policy role of the small area variations and physician practice style hypothesis. *Health Policy* 24(1):9-17.

Studnicki J. 1975. The minimization of travel effort as a delineating influence for urban hospital service areas. *International Journal of Health Services* 5(4):679-693.

Thomas JW, JR Griffith, and P Durance. 1979. *The specification of hospital service communities in a large metropolitan area.* Michigan Hospital Performance Measures Field Test, Technical Paper No. 5.

Wennberg JE. 1984. Dealing with medical practice variations: A proposal for action. *Health Affairs* 3(2):139-148.

Wennberg JE, and A Gittlesohn. 1973. Small area variations in health care delivery. *Science* 182:1102-1107.

Wennberg JE, A Gittelsohn, and N Shapiro. 1975. Health care delivery in Maine III: Evaluating the level of hospital performance. *Journal of the Maine Medical Association* 66(11):298-306.

Wilson P, and P Tedeschi. 1984. Community correlates of hospital use. *Health Services Research* 19(3):333-355.

Wright GE, and FS Marlor. 1990. *Alternative hospital market area definitions.* Deliverable No. Four, Final Report. Submitted to Prospective Payment Assessment Commission. Contract No. T-47540316.

Zwanziger J, and GA Melnick. 1988. The effects of hospital competition and the Medicare PPS program on hospital cost behavior in California. *Journal of Health Economics* 7:301-320.

Zwanziger J, GA Melnick, and JM Mann. 1990. Measures of hospital market structure: A review of the alternatives and a proposed approach. *Socioeconomic Planning Science* 24(2):81-95.

CHAPTER 8 CONTAGIOUS DISEASES

Adesina HO. 1984. The diffusion of cholera outside Ibadan City, Nigeria, 1971. *Social Science and Medicine* 18(5):421-428.

A strategic plan for the elimination of tuberculosis in the United States. 1989. *MMWR* 38:269-272.

Baker SR. 1979. The diffusion of high technology medical innovation: The computer tomography scanner example. *Social Science and Medicine* 13D:155-162.

Centers for Disease Control (CDC). 1990. HIV prevalence estimates and AIDS case projections for the United States: Report based upon a workshop. *MMWR* 39(RR-16):1-8,12-15.

Centers for Disease Control (CDC). 1988. HIV seroprevalence in migrant and seasonal farm workers—North Carolina, 1987. *MMWR* 37:517-519.

Centers for Disease Control (CDC). 1992. *HIV/AIDS Surveillance Report* January:1-22.

Centers for Disease Control (CDC). 1992. *HIV/AIDS Surveillance Report* July:1-18.

Centers for Disease Control (CDC). 1991a. The HIV/AIDS epidemic: The first 10 years. *MMWR* 40:357.

Centers for Disease Control and Prevention (CDC). 1993. Telephone communication with Press Office.

Centers for Disease Control. 1991b. *Tuberculosis statistics in the United States, 1989.* HHS Publication No. (CDC) 91-8322:73.

Centers for Disease Control. 1992. Update: Acquired immunodeficiency syndrome—United States, 1991. *MMWR* 41:462-468.

Ciesielski SD, JR Seed, DH Esposito, and N Hunter. 1991. The epidemiology of tuberculosis among North Carolina migrant farm workers. *Journal of the American Medical Association* 265(13):1715-19.

Cliff AD, and P Haggett. 1988. *Atlas of disease distributions: Analytic approaches to epidemiological data.* Oxford, UK: Basil Blackwell.

Cliff AD, P Haggett, and JK Ord. 1986. *Spatial aspects of influenza.* London: Pion.

Cliff AD, P Haggett, and DF Stroup. 1992. The geographic structure of measles epidemics in the northeastern United States. *American Journal of Epidemiology* 136(5):592-602.

Cohn SE, JE Mohr, JD Klein, CM van der Horst, and DJ Weber. 1992. *Migration of HIV-infected patients to North Carolina: An emerging rural phenomenon.* Chapel Hill, NC: North Carolina Rural Health Research Program, Cecil G. Sheps Center for Health Services Research.

Davis K, and J Stapleton. 1991. Migration to rural areas by HIV patients: Impact on HIV-related healthcare use. *Infection Control and Hospital Epidemiology* 12(9):540-43.

Dooley SW, WR Jarvis, WJ Martone, and DE Snider Jr. 1992. Multidrug-resistant tuberculosis. *Annals of Internal Medicine* 117(3):257-9.

Dubos R. 1965. *Man adapting.* New Haven, CT: Yale University Press.

Dy C. 1991. *The geography of AIDS in North Carolina.* Honors essay. Department of Geography, University of North Carolina at Chapel Hill.

Feinleib M, and AO Zarate, eds. 1992. Reconsidering age-adjustment procedures: Workshop proceedings. National Center for Health Statistics. *Vital Health Statistics* 4(29). DHHS Publication No. 93-1466. Washington, DC: US Government Printing Office.

Gardner LI Jr, JF Brundage, DS Burke, JG McNeil, R Visintine, and RN Miller. 1989. Evidence for spread of the human immuno-deficiency virus epidemic into low prevalence areas of the United States. *Journal of Acquired Immune Deficiency Syndromes* 2(6):521-532.

Gould PR. 1969. *Spatial diffusion.* Resource Paper No. 14. Washington, DC: Association of American Geographers.

Hennekens CH, and JE Buring. 1987. *Epidemiology in medicine.* Boston: Little Brown.

Jereb JA, GD Kelly, SW Dooley Jr, GM Cauthen, DE Snider Jr. 1991. Tuberculosis morbidity in the United States: Final data, 1990. *MMWR CDC Surveillance Summaries* 40(3):23-7.

Karon JM, and RL Berkelman. 1991. The geographic and ethnic diversity of AIDS incidence trends in homosexual/bisexual men in the United States. *Journal of Acquired Immune Deficiency Syndromes* 4(12):1179-89.

Migrant Health Task Force. 1991. North Carolina Farmworker Council. *The status of migrant health in North Carolina.* With research and draft preparation by the North Carolina Primary Health Care Association.

North Carolina Department of Labor. 1992. Division of Occupational Safety and Health, Bureau of Migrant Housing. *Migrant Housing Bulletin.* No. 2.

Patterson KD, and GF Pyle. 1983. The diffusion of influenza in sub-Saharan Africa during the 1918-1919 pandemic. *Social Science and Medicine* 17(17):1299-1307.

Pyle GF. 1986. *The diffusion of influenza: Patterns and paradigms.* Totowa, NJ: Rowan & Littlefield.

Pyle GF, and OJ Furuseth. 1992. The diffusion of AIDS and social deprivation in North Carolina. *The North Carolina Geographer* 1:1-10.

Shannon GW, GF Pyle, and RL Bashshur. 1991. *The geography of AIDS: Origins and course of an epidemic.* New York: Guilford Press.

St. Louis ME, GA Conway, CR Hayman, C Miller, LR Petersen, and TJ Dondero. 1991. Human immunodeficiency virus infection in disadvantaged adolescents: Findings from the US Job Corps. *Journal of the American Medical Association* 266(17):2387-91.

Sudre P, G ten Dam, and A Kochi. 1992. Tuberculosis: A global overview of the situation today. *Bulletin of the World Health Organization* 70(2):149-59.

Thomas R. 1992. *Geomedical systems: Intervention and control.* London: Routledge.

US Bureau of the Census. 1991. Census of population and housing, 1990: Summary tape 1A. Washington, DC.

US Geological Survey. 1988. The geographic names information system: The national geographic names data base. Washington, DC.

Verghese A, SL Berk, and F Sarubbi. 1989. Urbs in rure: Human immunodeficiency virus infection in rural Tennessee. *Journal of Infectious Diseases* 160(6):1051-5.

CHAPTER 9 EVALUATING CLUSTERS OF ADVERSE HEALTH OUTCOMES

Aldrich TE. 1990. *CLUSTER: User's manual for software to assist with investigations of rare health events*. Atlanta, GA: Agency for Toxic Substances and Disease Registries.

Aldrich TE, DE Atkinson, A Hines, and CG Smith. 1990. The establishment of a population-based cancer registry for North Carolina. *North Carolina Medical Journal* 51(2):107-112.

Aldrich TE, J Lindsey, and P Morris. 1991. *Evaluation of cancer cluster reports in North Carolina*. CHES Studies. State of North Carolina, Department of Environment, Health, and Natural Resources, No. 56.

Aldrich TE, RE Meyer, J Qualters, and DE Atkinson. 1989. Rare health events as sentinels of environmental contamination. In: *Proceedings: 1989 public health conference on records and statistics*. DHHS Publication No. 90-1214, pp. 323-326.

Aldrich TE, CC Wilson, and CE Easterly. 1985. Population surveillance for rare health events. In: *Proceedings: 1985 Public Health Conference on Records and Statistics*. DHHS Publication No. 86-1214, pp. 215-220.

Armenian HK. 1991. Case investigation in epidemiology. *American Journal of Epidemiology* 134(10):1067-1072.

Barton DE, FN David, and M Merrington. 1965. A criterion for testing contagion in time and space. *Annals of Human Genetics* 29:97-101.

Bender AP, AN Williams, RA Johnson, and HG Jagger. 1990. Appropriate public health responses to clusters: The art of being responsibly responsible. *American Journal of Epidemiology* 132:S48-S52.

Centers for Disease Control (CDC). 1990. Guidelines for investigating clusters of health events. *MMWR* 39(No. RR-11).

Doll R. 1981. Relevance of epidemiology to policies for the prevention of cancer. *Journal of Occupational Medicine* 23:601-9.

Fiore BJ, LP Haranhan, and HA Anderson. 1990. State health department response to disease cluster reports: A protocol for investigation. *American Journal of Epidemiology* 132:S14-S22.

Gibbons RD, and DC Clark. 1992. Letter to the editor. *American Journal of Epidemiology* 135(11):1310-1314.

Glaser SL. 1990. Spatial clustering of Hodgkin's Disease in the San Francisco Bay Area. *American Journal of Epidemiology* 132:S167-S177.

Glasser JH. 1985. *Health statistics surveillance systems for hazardous substance disposal.* Proceedings from the 1985 Public Health Conference on Records and Statistics. DHHS Publication No. 86-1214, pp. 221-224.

Glick B. 1979. The spatial autocorrelation of cancer mortality. *Social Science and Medicine* 13D:123-130.

Grimson RC, KC Wang, and PWC Johnson. 1981. Searching for hierarchical clusters of disease, spatial patterns of sudden infant death syndrome. *Social Science and Medicine* 15D(2):287-93.

Hardy RJ, GD Schroeder, SP Cooper, PA Buffler, HM Prichard, and M Crane. 1990. A surveillance system for assessing health effects from hazardous exposures. *American Journal of Epidemiology* 132(1 suppl):S32-42.

Hartigan JA. 1975. *Clustering algorithms.* NY: John Wiley & Sons.

Hatch MC, S Wallenstein, J Beyea, JW Nieves, and M Susser. 1991. Cancer rates after the Three Mile Island nuclear accident and proximity of residence to the plant. *American Journal of Public Health* 81(6):719-724.

Heath CW. 1990. Author's reply to thymic function and leukemia. CA: *A Journal for Clinicians* 40:319-20.

Hill GB, CC Spicer, and JAC Weatherall. 1968. The computer surveillance for congenital malformations. *British Medical Bulletin* 24:215-218.

Houk VN, and SB Thacker. 1987. Registries: One way to assess environmental hazards. *Health and the Environment Digest* 1:5-6.

Knox EG. 1964. The detection of space-time interactions. *Applied Statistics* 13:25-29.

Monson RR. 1990. Editorial comment: Epidemiology and exposure to electromagnetic fields. *American Journal of Epidemiology* 131:774-75.

Naus JI. 1982. Approximations for distributions of scan statistics. *Journal of the American Statistical Association* 77:177-83.

Neutra RR. 1990. Counterpoint from a cluster buster. *American Journal of Epidemiology* 132(1):1-8.

Ohno Y, and K Aoki. 1981. Cancer deaths by city and county in Japan (1969-1971): A test of significance for geographic clusters of disease. *Social Science and Medicine* 15D:251-258.

Parzen E. 1960. *Modern probability theory and its application.* New York: John Wiley and Sons.

Riise T, and MR Klauber. 1992. Relationship between the degree of individual space-time clustering and age at onset of disease among multiple sclerosis patients. *International Journal of Epidemiology* 21(3):528-532.

Rodrigues LC, Marshall T, Murphy M, and Osmond C. 1992. Space time clustering of births in SIDS: Do perinatal infections play a role? *International Journal of Epidemiology* 21(4):714-719.

Ross A, and S Davis. 1990. Point pattern analysis of the spatial proximity of residences prior to diagnosis of persons with

Hodgkin's disease. *American Journal of Epidemiology* 132(1): S53-S62.

Rothman KJ. 1990. A sobering start to the cluster busters' conference. *American Journal of Epidemiology* 132:S6-S13.

Rothwell CJ, CB Hamilton, and PE Leaverton. 1991. Identification of sentinel health events as indicators of environmental contamination. *Environmental Health Perspectives* 94:261-63.

Ruckelshous WD. 1984. Risk in a free society. *Risk Analysis* 4:157-62.

Schneider D, Greenberg MR, Donaldson MH, and Choi D. 1993. Cancer clusters: The importance of monitoring multiple geographic scales. *Social Science and Medicine* 37(6):753-759.

Shafer S. 1980. Mapping bone cancer death rates in pennsylvania counties. *Social Science and Medicine* 14D:11-15.

Thacker SB. 1989. Time-space clusters: The public health dilemma. *Health and Environment Digest* 3:4-5.

Thacker SB, and RL Berkelman. 1988. Public health surveillance in the United States. *Epidemiologic Reviews* 10:164-190.

Verhasselt Y. 1977. Notes on geography and cancer. *Social Science and Medicine* 11:745-748.

Wallenstein S. 1980. A test for detection of clustering over time. *American Journal of Epidemiology* 11:367-72.

Index

About the Contributors

Author Listing

(in alphabetical order by last name)

Don Albert, MA, Doctoral Student, Department of Geography, and Graduate Research Assistant/Cartographer, North Carolina Rural Health Research Program, Cecil G. Sheps Center for Health Services Research, University of North Carolina at Chapel Hill

Timothy E. Aldrich, PhD, Adjunct Assistant Professor, Department of Epidemiology, University of North Carolina at Chapel Hill

Susan E. Cohn, MD, Health Services Research Post-Doctoral Fellow, North Carolina Rural Health Research Program, Cecil G. Sheps Center for Health Services Research, University of North Carolina at Chapel Hill

Susan I. DesHarnais, PhD, Associate Professor, Department of Health Policy and Administration, University of North Carolina at Chapel Hill

John Florin, PhD, Associate Professor and Chair, Department of Geography, University of North Carolina at Chapel Hill

Lise K. Fondren, MA, Policy Associate, Cecil G. Sheps Center for Health Services Research

Wilbert M. Gesler, PhD, Associate Professor, Department of Geography, University of North Carolina at Chapel Hill

Anne M. Jacobs, MHA, Doctoral Candidate, Department of Health Policy and Administration, and Health Services Research Pre-Doctoral Fellow, Cecil G. Sheps Center for Health Services Research, University of North Carolina at Chapel Hill

Thomas R. Konrad, PhD, Research Associate Professor, Department of Social Medicine and Director, Program on Health Professionals, Cecil G. Sheps Center for Health Services Research, University of North Carolina at Chapel Hill

John Lowe, MS, Adjunct Lecturer and Doctoral Candidate, School of Urban Planning and Policy, The University of Illinois at Chicago

Melinda Meade, PhD, Professor, Department of Geography, University of North Carolina at Chapel Hill

Adrian Menapace, MSPH, Graduate Research Assistant, Department of Health Policy and Administration, University of North Carolina at Chapel Hill

Peter S. Millard, MD, Health Services Research Post-Doctoral Fellow, North Carolina Rural Health Research Program, Cecil G. Sheps Center for Health Services Research, University of North Carolina at Chapel Hill

Laura Moorhead, MA, Doctoral Candidate, Department of Geography, and Graduate Research Assistant, North Carolina Rural Health Research Program, Cecil G. Sheps Center for Health Services Research, University of North Carolina at Chapel Hill

Diana N. Osborne, BA, Information and Communications Specialist, North Carolina Rural Health Research Program, Cecil G. Sheps Center for Health Services Research, University of North Carolina at Chapel Hill

Forrest Pommerenke, MD, Director, Early Detection Branch, Division of Cancer Prevention and Control, National Cancer Institute, National Institutes of Health, US Department of Health and Human Services

Thomas C. Ricketts, III, PhD, Assistant Professor, Department of Health Policy and Administration and Director, North Carolina Rural Health Research Program, Cecil G. Sheps Center for Health Services Research, University of North Carolina at Chapel Hill

Lucy A. Savitz, MBA, Doctoral Candidate, Department of Health Policy and Administration, and Graduate Research Assistant, North Carolina Rural Health Research Program, Cecil G. Sheps Center for Health Services Research, University of North Carolina at Chapel Hill

Kit N. Simpson, DrPH, Assistant Professor, Department of Health Policy and Administration, University of North Carolina at Chapel Hill

Peggy Wittie, MAG, Doctoral Student, Department of Geography, University of North Carolina at Chapel Hill